Evaluation of the Surgical Margin

Editors

JOSHUA E. LUBEK
KELLY R. MAGLIOCCA

ORAL AND MAXILLOFACIAL SURGERY CLINICS OF NORTH AMERICA

www.oralmaxsurgery.theclinics.com

Consulting Editor
RICHARD H. HAUG

August 2017 • Volume 29 • Number 3

ELSEVIER

1600 John F. Kennedy Boulevard • Suite 1800 • Philadelphia, Pennsylvania, 19103-2899

http://www.oralmaxsurgery.theclinics.com

ORAL AND MAXILLOFACIAL SURGERY CLINICS OF NORTH AMERICA Volume 29, Number 3
August 2017 ISSN 1042-3699, ISBN-13: 978-0-323-53247-1

Editor: John Vassallo; j.vassallo@elsevier.com
Developmental Editor: Colleen Dietzler

Oral and Maxillofacial Surgery Clinics of North America (ISSN 1042-3699) is published quarterly by Elsevier Inc., 360 Park Avenue South, New York, NY 10010-1710. Months of issue are February, May, August, and November. Business and Editorial Offices: 1600 John F. Kennedy Blvd., Suite 1800, Philadelphia, PA 19103-2899. Periodicals postage paid at New York, NY and additional mailing offices. Subscription prices are $385.00 per year for US individuals, $653.00 per year for US institutions, $100.00 per year for US students and residents, $455.00 per year for Canadian individuals, $783.00 per year for Canadian institutions, $520.00 per year for international individuals, $783.00 per year for international institutions and $235.00 per year for Canadian and foreign students/residents. To receive student/resident rate, orders must be accompanied by name or affiliated institution, date of term, and the *signature* of program/residency coordinator on institution letterhead. Orders will be billed at individual rate until proof of status is received. Foreign air speed delivery is included in all *Clinics* subscription prices. All prices are subject to change without notice. **POSTMASTER:** Send address changes to *Oral and Maxillofacial Surgery Clinics of North America,* Elsevier Periodicals **Customer Service, 11830 Westline Industrial Drive, St. Louis, MO 63146. Tel: 1-800-654-2452 (U.S. and Canada); 314-447-8871 (outside U.S. and Canada). Fax: 314-447-8029. E-mail: journals customerservice-usa@elsevier.com (for print support); journalsonlinesupport-usa@elsevier.com (for online support).**

Reprints. For copies of 100 or more, of articles in this publication, please contact the Commercial Reprints Department, Elsevier Inc., 360 Park Avenue South, New York, NY 10010-1710. Tel.: 212-633-3874; Fax: 212-633-3820; Email: reprints@elsevier.com.

Oral and Maxillofacial Surgery Clinics of North America is covered in *MEDLINE/PubMed* (*Index Medicus*), *Science Citation Index Expanded* (*SciSearch®*), *Journal Citation Reports/Science Edition*, and *Current Contents®/Clinical Medicine*.

Printed in the United States of America.

Contributors

CONSULTING EDITOR

RICHARD H. HAUG, DDS
Professor and Chief, Oral Maxillofacial Surgery,
Carolinas Medical Center, Charlotte, North
Carolina

EDITORS

JOSHUA E. LUBEK, DDS, MD, FACS
Associate Professor and Fellowship Director,
Oral-Head & Neck Surgery/Microvascular
Surgery, Department of Oral and Maxillofacial
Surgery, University of Maryland, Baltimore,
Maryland

KELLY R. MAGLIOCCA, DDS, MPH
Assistant Professor, Oral, Head and Neck
Pathology, Department of Pathology and
Laboratory Medicine, Emory University,
Atlanta, Georgia

AUTHORS

R. BRYAN BELL, MD, DDS, FACS, FACD
Medical Director, Providence Oral, Head and
Neck Cancer Program, Consultant, Head
and Neck Institute, Investigator, Earle A.
Chiles Research Institute, Department of
Pathology, Providence Cancer Center,
Providence Portland Medical Center, Portland,
Oregon

STEVE CALDRONEY, DDS, MD
Fellow in Head and Neck/Microvascular
Surgery, Department of Oral and Maxillofacial
Surgery, University of Maryland, Baltimore,
Maryland

ERIC R. CARLSON, DMD, MD, FACS
Professor and Kelly L. Krahwinkel Chairman,
Director, Oral and Maxillofacial Surgery
Residency Program, Director, Oral/Head
and Neck Oncologic Surgery Fellowship
Program, Department of Oral and
Maxillofacial Surgery, University of
Tennessee Medical Center, University of

Tennessee Cancer Institute, Knoxville,
Tennessee

DAVID J. CLARK, PhD
Postdoctoral Fellow, Department of Pathology,
Johns Hopkins Medical Institute, Baltimore,
Maryland

DONITA DYALRAM, DDS, MD, FACS
Assistant Professor, Department of Oral and
Maxillofacial Surgery, University of Maryland,
Baltimore, Maryland

**SEAN P. EDWARDS, MD, DDS, FACS,
FRCD(C)**
James R Hayward Endowed Professor of
Oral and Maxillofacial Surgery, Clinical
Associate Professor of Dentistry, Associate
Professor of Surgery, Director, Oral and
Maxillofacial Surgery Residency Program,
University of Michigan, Chief, Pediatric
Maxillofacial Surgery, C.S. Mott Children's
Hospital, Michigan Medicine, Ann Arbor,
Michigan

RUI FERNANDES, MD, DMD
Program Director, Head and Neck Oncologic
Surgery and Microvascular Fellowship, Chief,
Division of Head and Neck Surgery, Associate
Chair, Department of Oral and Maxillofacial
Surgery, University of Florida Health Science
Center, Jacksonville, University of Florida
College of Medicine, Jacksonville, Florida

**NASEEM GHAZALI, MSc, DOHNS, FDSRCS,
FRCS(OMFS)**
Fellow, Oncology/Microvascular Surgery,
University of Maryland Dental School,
University of Maryland Medical Center,
Greenbaum Cancer Center, Baltimore,
Maryland

ARUN GOPINATH, MD
Assistant Professor, Director, Head and
Neck Pathology, Department of Pathology
and Laboratory Medicine, University of
Florida College of Medicine, University
of Florida, Jacksonville, Jacksonville,
Florida

JONATHON HEATH, MD
Assistant Professor, Department of Pathology,
University of Maryland School of Medicine,
Baltimore, Maryland

JOSEPH I. HELMAN, DMD
Professor, Department of Oral and
Maxillofacial Surgery, University of Michigan,
Ann Arbor, Michigan

ANTONIA KOLOKYTHAS, DDS, MSc, FACS
Head and Program Director, Department of Oral
and Maxillofacial Surgery, Strong Memorial
Hospital, University of Rochester-Eastman
Institute for Oral Health, Rochester, New York

JOSHUA E. LUBEK, DDS, MD, FACS
Associate Professor and Fellowship Director,
Oral-Head & Neck Surgery/Microvascular
Surgery, Department of Oral and Maxillofacial
Surgery, University of Maryland, Baltimore,
Maryland

KELLY R. MAGLIOCCA, DDS, MPH
Assistant Professor, Oral, Head and Neck
Pathology, Department of Pathology and
Laboratory Medicine, Emory University,
Atlanta, Georgia

RAAFAT F. MAKARY, MBBCh (MD), PhD
Associate Professor, Director, Soft Tissue
Pathology, Neuropathology and Autopsy
Services, Department of Pathology and
Laboratory Medicine, University of Florida
College of Medicine, University of Florida,
Jacksonville, Jacksonville, Florida

LI MAO, MD
Former Professor and Chair, Department of
Oncology and Diagnostic Sciences, University
of Maryland School of Dentistry, Baltimore,
Maryland

MICHAEL R. MARKIEWICZ, DDS, MPH, MD
Fellow, Head and Neck Oncologic and
Microvascular Surgery, Division of Head Neck
Surgery, Department of Oral and Maxillofacial
Surgery, University of Florida Health Science
Center, Jacksonville, Division of Surgical
Oncology, University of Florida College of
Medicine, Jacksonville, Florida

JAMES MICHAEL McCOY, DDS, FACS
Professor, Departments of Oral and
Maxillofacial Surgery, Pathology and
Radiology, University of Tennessee Medical
Center, Knoxville, Tennessee

LINDSAY MONTAGUE, DMD
Assistant Professor, Division Head Oral
Pathology, Department of Oral & Maxillofacial
Surgery and Pathology, School of Dentistry,
University of Mississippi Medical Center,
Jackson, Mississippi

ROBERT A. ORD, MS, MBA, FACS, FRCS
Chairman/Professor, Department of Oral and
Maxillofacial Surgery, University of Maryland
Dental School, University of Maryland Medical
Center, Greenebaum Cancer Center,
Baltimore, Maryland

MOHAMMED QAISI, DMD, MD, FACS
Program Director, Division of Oral &
Maxillofacial Surgery, Attending Physician,
Division of Otolaryngology, John H. Stroger,
Jr. Hospital of Cook County, Chicago, Illinois

ERIC RINGER, DDS
Senior Resident, Department of Oral and
Maxillofacial Surgery, University of
Rochester-Eastman Institute for Oral Health,
Rochester, New York

ANDREW SALAMA, DDS, MD
Residency Director, Department of Oral and Maxillofacial Surgery, Boston Medical Center, Assistant Professor, Boston University School of Dental Medicine, Boston, Massachusetts

MICHAEL SHAPIRO, DDS, MA
Chief Resident, Department of Oral and Maxillofacial Surgery, Boston Medical Center, Boston, Massachusetts

FELIX W. SIM, MBBS, BDS, MFDS(Eng), FRACDS(OMS)
Fellow, Head and Neck Oncology and Microvascular Reconstructive Surgery, Head and Neck Institute, Department of Pathology, Providence Cancer Center, Providence Portland Medical Center, Portland, Oregon

HONG D. XIAO, MD, PhD
Head and Neck Pathologist, Department of Pathology, Providence Cancer Center, Providence Portland Medical Center, Portland, Oregon

Contents

the treatment plan. This article focuses on methods of evaluation of the bone margin in the preoperative and intraoperative setting, discussing the implications for prognostic, staging, and reconstructive methods.

Bone Margin Analysis for Benign Odontogenic Tumors

Eric Ringer and Antonia Kolokythas

With the potential exception of the case of ameloblastoma, information relevant to the exact tumor–bone interface and extent of bone invasion by the commonly encountered odontogenic tumors is lacking. These tumors are rare. Treatment rendered varies significantly. Although commonly accepted practices are recommended, scientific evidence is relatively lacking. Prospective multicenter studies from tertiary treatment centers are required for evidence-based guidelines. Until studies are available, the proposed linear bone resection margin for odontogenic tumors and the evaluation of its adequacy in tumor eradication will be based on the limited data available.

Bone Margin Analysis for Osteonecrosis and Osteomyelitis of the Jaws

Mohammed Qaisi and Lindsay Montague

Bone margin analysis in cases of osteomyelitis, osteoradionecrosis, and medication-related osteonecrosis of the jaw is a controversial topic. There is little evidence to guide treatment and the interpretation of bone margin results. This article examines the significance of margin status and any possible effect on progression of the disease process. A review of various treatment adjuncts used for intraoperative margin analysis during removal of affected tissue is provided. Literature on the role of imaging is also discussed with regards to treatment planning for surgical resection. The histology of the three separate entities including the approach to surgical and pathologic evaluation of margins is also discussed.

Margin Analysis: Malignant Salivary Gland Neoplasms of the Head and Neck

Robert A. Ord and Naseem Ghazali

There are no established protocols for the optimum surgical margin required for salivary gland malignancies. Factors including histologic diagnosis and TNM stage have been shown to be important in prognosis and survival outcome and mandate special consideration of margin size. Salivary cancers are treated differently at different anatomic sites, and different histologic types show a propensity for major or minor glands. Low-grade malignancies are treated with soft tissue margins of 1 cm or less. The facial nerve is preserved unless infiltrated and encased. Adenoid cystic carcinoma and carcinoma ex pleomorphic adenoma require more complex planning to obtain negative margins.

Margins for Benign Salivary Gland Neoplasms of the Head and Neck

Eric R. Carlson and James Michael McCoy

The proper ablation of any neoplasm of the head and neck requires the inclusion of linear and anatomic barrier margins surrounding the neoplasm. Extirpative surgery of the major and minor salivary glands is certainly no exception to this surgical principle. To this end, the selection and execution of the most appropriate ablative surgical procedure for a major or minor benign salivary gland neoplasm is an essential exercise in oral and maxillofacial surgery. Of equal importance is the intraoperative identification and preservation of the pseudocapsule surrounding the benign neoplasm. This article reviews these important elements specifically related to ablative surgery of benign neoplasms of the parotid, submandibular and minor salivary glands with strict attention to observed nomenclature.

This article focuses only on margin analysis of the cutaneous malignancy of the skin. It discusses basal cell carcinoma, squamous cell carcinoma, and cutaneous melanoma. The management of the neck and distant disease are beyond the scope of this article, but it answers what is the appropriate surgical margin when excising these skin tumors, whether frozen sections are accurate for the analysis of these tumors, and treatment algorithm and rationale for a positive resection margin.

Head and neck sarcomas are rare but are associated with significant morbidity/mortality and management difficulties. These tumors are best managed in a multidisciplinary setting. Open or core biopsy is essential for histologic diagnosis and grading. Complete surgical tumor resection with negative margins at the first attempt is the best chance for potential cure. In most patients, except those with small resectable low-grade lesions, adjuvant radiotherapy and chemotherapy are added to maximize local control with variable results. Resection margins effect on recurrence rate and treatment modalities in selective types of head and neck sarcomas are discussed in this article.

Neoplasms of the head and neck constitute a broad spectrum of benign and malignant entities. When treatment involves resection, assessment of the surgical margins represents an important component of the pathologic examination. Margin status is an important indicator of a complete surgical resection. The ability to generalize conclusions such as 'safe distance' measurements from work performed mSCCa or cutaneous malignancy to other types of neoplasms in the head and neck region seems limited. This article reviews conditions and considerations for reliable margin assessment and interpretation.

Microvascular reconstruction of ablative defects has become a mainstay of contemporary management of head and neck cancer patients. These techniques offer myriad tissue options that vary in character, volume, and components and have vastly improved the esthetic and functional outcomes achieved in this patient population. Although consensus exists regarding the reliability and functional and esthetic benefits of free tissue transfer, the same cannot be said for oncologic outcomes. The increase in resources required for the routine use of free tissue transfer has led to asking this question—Do vascularized free flaps allow for increased surgical margins and improvements in oncologic outcomes?

ORAL AND MAXILLOFACIAL SURGERY CLINICS OF NORTH AMERICA

THE CLINICS ARE NOW AVAILABLE ONLINE!
Access your subscription at:
www.theclinics.com

Introduction

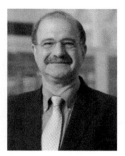

Joseph I. Helman, DMD

The instructions for cancer operations by the accomplished surgeon Galen in the second century AD were to "make accurate incisions surrounding the entire tumor as not to leave a single root."

Progress in the management of cancer surgery wasn't very significant until the mid-19th century when Dr Rudolf Virchow published his book, *Cellular Pathology*, in 1958, which is considered the pioneer work of modern Pathology.

Both Galen and Virchow believed in the surgical management of specific malignant tumors, which should be resected with *clean margins.*

Dr Joshua Lubek and Dr Kelly Magliocca have both edited an outstanding issue for the *Oral and Maxillofacial Surgery Clinics of North America* on the Evaluation of the Surgical Margin, addressing subjects like molecular markers of the margins, the challenges of the bone margin, and the bridging between pathology and surgery in order to improve the communication and understanding between the two professional disciplines.

The authors of each article represent the highest level of academic integrity, honesty, knowledge, and critical thinking. They have a commitment to share their experience with their peers in a selfless fashion in order to improve education without biased thoughts and with scientific rigor.

This issue fulfills the objective of scientific curiosity and education. This brings me to a different subject: Education is eternal, immortal. It lives forever, transmitted from generation to generation. It enhances knowledge and understanding. In this specific case, it makes me incredibly proud. Both of the editors, Kelly Magliocca and Josh Lubek, were trainees at the University of Michigan while I was leading the Department of Oral and Maxillofacial Surgery. I had the unique opportunity to provide them with professional guidance and personal advice. They are part of my extended family, and when I see their achievements, I do smile with happiness.

There is no greater satisfaction in academic life than to see your former interns, residents, and fellows succeed and become the leaders and the best!

Thank you for becoming who you are now!

Joseph I. Helman, DMD
Department of Oral and Maxillofacial Surgery
University of Michigan
1500 East Medical Center Drive
Towsley Center–Room G1113
Ann Arbor, MI 48109, USA

E-mail address:
jihelman@med.umich.edu

Oral Maxillofacial Surg Clin N Am 29 (2017) xi
http://dx.doi.org/10.1016/j.coms.2017.06.006
1042-3699/17/© 2017 Published by Elsevier Inc.

Preface

Evaluation of the Surgical Margin: An Interdisciplinary Approach

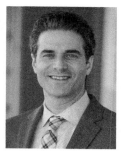 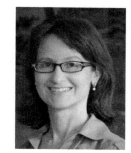

Joshua E. Lubek, DDS, MD, FACS   Kelly R. Magliocca, DDS, MPH
Editors

The aim of this issue of *Oral and Maxillofacial Surgery Clinics of North America* is to provide an interdisciplinary perspective on the study of the surgical margin as it relates to a spectrum of disease processes affecting the head and neck. There is much debate as to what is considered a "negative" surgical margin in the oncology literature. The reported final margin status will ultimately affect the clinical decision of the treating surgeon with regards to re-treatment or recommendation for adjuvant therapies. To improve accuracy and clarity of the final margin status, both the surgeon and the pathologist must understand the interdisciplinary perspective, particularly limitations of surgical technique and/or pathologic examination as it relates to the surgical margin.

The Guest Editors wish to acknowledge and thank all of the authors for their time, expertise, and contributions in the writing of this issue of *Oral and Maxillofacial Surgery Clinics of North America* dedicated to the study of the surgical margin. A special thanks to John Vassallo, Colleen Dietzler, and the Elsevier team for their patience, guidance, and the opportunity to present this important topic and foster future discussion and collaborative efforts aimed at enhancing quality patient care.

Joshua E. Lubek, DDS, MD, FACS
Oral Head & Neck Surgery/Microvascular Surgery
Department of Oral and Maxillofacial Surgery
University of Maryland
University of Maryland Oral and
Maxillofacial Surgery Associates
650 West Baltimore Street, Room #1401
Baltimore, MD 21201, USA

Kelly R. Magliocca, DDS, MPH
Department of Pathology and Laboratory
Medicine
Emory University
Emory Pathology and Laboratory Medicine
1364 Clifton Road Northeast, Room H183
Atlanta, GA 30322, USA

E-mail addresses:
jlubek@umaryland.edu (J.E. Lubek)
kmagliocca@emory.edu (K.R. Magliocca)

Oral Maxillofacial Surg Clin N Am 29 (2017) xiii
http://dx.doi.org/10.1016/j.coms.2017.05.003
1042-3699/17/© 2017 Published by Elsevier Inc.

Understanding the Surgical Margin
A Molecular Assessment

David J. Clark, PhD[a], Li Mao, MD[b],*

KEYWORDS

- Molecular margins • Head and neck malignancy • p53 mutation • Field cancerization

KEY POINTS

- The theories of minimal residual cancer and field cancerization can help to explain reasons for tumor recurrence despite negative histologic surgical margins.
- Histologically benign tissue adjacent to premalignant lesions have genomic alterations.
- Molecular information can help improve outcomes in surgical margin analysis not able to be detected on hematoxylin and eosin frozen section.
- Human papillomavirus (HPV)-negative tumors display a twofold increase in mutations relative to HPV-positive tumors.

SURGICAL RESECTION OF HEAD AND NECK CANCERS

Head and neck cancer is a broad term for malignancies developing in the epithelial cells lining the oral cavity, pharynx, and larynx. In the United States, there are estimated 59,000 new incidences of head and neck squamous cell carcinoma (HNSCC) diagnosed, with approximately 12,000 related deaths, in 2015 alone.[1] On diagnosis, factors including tumor location, staging, and the patient's age and health status are assessed to determine the best modality of treatment for individual patients, with most treated via surgery.[2] The central tenet of surgical resection in HNSCC is the complete removal of the tumor, wherein, a surgeon will resect the gross tumor in addition to surrounding tissues that may contain invading cancer cells. Histologic assessment by a pathologist is used to determine if cancer cells are detectable at the edge of the resection, which would be indicative of a positive surgical margin (presenting tumor cells). With a correlation between evidence of a positive margin in resected surgical samples

and tumor recurrence, as well as a decreased survival, surgeons may elect to remove additional surrounding tissues until a negative margin is obtained.[2,3] A confounding aspect of surgical resection in HNSCC is the limited anatomic area of the head and neck, where aggressive surgical efforts to remove cancerous regions and obtain a negative surgical margin may reduce the functionality of various organs (ie, tongue, larynx), as well as significantly impacting the postoperative quality of life for the patient.

INCORPORATING MOLECULAR SURGICAL MARGINS IN HEAD AND NECK CANCER

Accurate histologic assessment of margins in HNSCC surgical resections is vital; however, the variety of anatomic sites and respective differences in surgical approach results in a lack of standardization regarding the definition of an adequate margin. Resulting from this variability, histopathological examination within HNSCC can be subjective, and the classification of disease severity (ie, moderate dysplasia vs in situ, or

[a] Department of Pathology, Johns Hopkins Medical Institute, 400 North Broadway, Baltimore, MD 21231, USA;
[b] Department of Oncology and Diagnostic Sciences, University of Maryland School of Dentistry, 650 West Baltimore Street, Baltimore, MD 21201, USA
* Corresponding author.
E-mail address: umbmao@gmail.com

Oral Maxillofacial Surg Clin N Am 29 (2017) 245–258
http://dx.doi.org/10.1016/j.coms.2017.03.002
1042-3699/17/© 2017 Elsevier Inc. All rights reserved.

severe dysplasia) by one pathologist may conflict with another.[4] When members of the American Head and Neck Society were surveyed concerning the classification of margins containing carcinoma in situ or dysplasia, most considered the former to be a positive margin, but not the latter.[5] The lack of uniform criterion in assessing the surgical margin may result in residual disease, which has severe consequences in terms of recurrence and overall patient survival, and it becomes evident that despite efforts to define the adequate surgical margin in HNSCC, histologic examination alone appears to be insufficient.

It has been well-established that cumulative genetic alterations facilitate the progression of premalignant lesions into HNSCC.[6] However, in premalignant lesions, the genetic alterations incurred may not result in morphologic changes, thus histologic examination alone may be inadequate in accurately defining the extent of disease.[7] Furthermore, certain differentiation agents may convert dysplastic lesions to "normal-looking" tissues histologically and therefore masking their underlying genetic alterations.[8] The inclusion of molecular characteristics into surgical margin analysis may not only yield a more sensitive and accurate assessment of the cells in these margins, but may also provide insight into their impacts to patients' postoperative prognosis. This concept of the "molecular surgical margin" (MSM) is advantageous, as it integrates recent advances in our understanding of head and neck carcinogenesis, while also retaining the established methodology of histopathology. This multidisciplinary approach may facilitate the development of a uniform criterion for defining the surgical margin, which will likely result in a reduced recurrence rate and improved overall patient survival.

UNDERSTANDING HEAD AND NECK SQUAMOUS CELL CARCINOMA RECURRENCE

The most significant metric regarding the success of surgical resection in HNSCC is the occurrence of disease relapse. One study reported that patients whose surgical resection met the respective criteria as satisfactory margins experienced a 12% recurrence rate at the primary tumor site, with patients displaying advanced disease having a higher rate of recurrence,[9] whereas others have suggested that despite histologic negative margin, a recurrence rate involving all sites could be as high as 30%.[10] Traditionally, a local recurrence is defined as the occurrence of another carcinoma less than 2 cm from the site of the initial resected carcinoma within a 3-year period. This definition was meant to distinguish local recurrence from second primary tumors (SPT), which were first defined by Warren and Gates[11] in 1932 as being a distinct, nonmetastatic malignancy, with the additional clinical criteria of occurring more than 2 cm from the initial anatomic site and diagnosed at least 3 years later being included.[12]

There are two theoretic explanations regarding the incidence of disease recurrence in HNSCC after surgical intervention. One theory involves the concept of minimal residual cancer (MRC), whereby a small number cancer cells, undetected by the pathologist examination of the surgical margin, remain and develop into a malignancy. A second theory of recurrence involves the concept of "field cancerization" first proposed by Slaughter and colleagues,[13] whereby after extensive histologic examination of oral cancers, the investigators summarized several observations: (1) oral and oropharyngeal cancer develops in multifocal regions of premalignant cells, (2) atypical tissue surrounds the tumor, (3) oral and oropharyngeal cancer is composed of multiple, independent lesions, and (4) the persistence of abnormal tissues gives rise to SPT and local recurrence. These two concepts of disease recurrence not only relate distinct mechanisms of cancer relapse, but may also impact the choice of therapeutic intervention.[14] Recurrences based on MRC theory may be treated by a combination of re-resection and postoperative radiotherapy. In contrast, treatment for recurrences due to field cancerization may be treated as a primary tumor with expanded fields containing premalignant cells. As both concepts relating to recurrence are related to the inadequacy of histologic assessment, additional methods that expand beyond macroscopic-based evidence need to be explored.

Incorporating molecular information into the analysis would not only provide more sensitive and specific determination of residue tumor cells, but also enable the detection of the "defected" field that cannot be histologically defined, and therefore allow a better understanding of disease progression and the basis of tumor recurrence. As observed in other cancer types, the accumulation of genetic alterations facilitates the transforming of a normal squamous epithelial cell into a cancer cell, and this transition is referred to as multistep carcinogenesis.[15,16] As described by Califano and colleagues,[16] the number of genetic alterations observed are in parallel with the level of malignancy presented in histologic examination. Furthermore, it was shown that even histologically benign tissues, adjacent to precancerous lesions, have acquired genomic alterations. In fact, it was revealed that these fields can have a fairly large diameter, with one study observing a "defected" field greater than 7 cm, which included genetic alterations in histologically normal mucosa.[17] Using two, distinct genetic markers, this latter study showed that several patients harbored first and second tumors that appeared to be clonal in origin, whereas others displayed first and second tumors that appeared genetically independent of one another. This observation indicates that the traditional criterion used to define local recurrence and SPTs may need revision (**Table 1**). With the knowledge that the "defected" field can be fairly large, one cannot accurately determine that a second tumor found more than 2 cm away is, in fact, a distinct, independent malignancy by histology alone, and instead, the molecular profile of each tumor should be assessed. In doing so, we may better define and differentiate first and SPTs, while also clarifying local recurrence occurring as a result of MRC, or a premalignant lesion not detected macroscopically in the field. Toward this end, the revised definition of local recurrence may include the previous criterion of the occurrence of another carcinoma less than 2 cm from the site of the initial resected carcinoma within a 3-year period, and the additional criteria that the new carcinoma displays an identical molecular pattern as the initial tumor. An SPT would be described as a new carcinoma occurring more than 2 cm from the initial anatomic site diagnosed at least 3 years later, and displaying a distinct molecular pattern from the initial tumor, indicating that the second carcinoma developed independently of the first. Finally, for "new" tumors that would arise in an anatomic region near the initial carcinoma, but displaying a similar molecular pattern, the classification as second field tumors (SFT) would be more accurate.[17] SFTs would be reflective of the biological impact of field cancerization,

in which a field of preneoplastic cells adjacent to the gross tumor share a similar molecular fingerprint, but develop into a malignancy after subsequent separate genomic events.

SURGICAL MARGIN MOLECULAR MARKERS

Tumorigenesis is a multistep process, in which early genetic events accumulate and eventually drive the progression of a normal cell toward a malignant phenotype.[18] In HNSCC, early events associated with genomic instability, including mutations and amplifications, are indicative of loss of heterozygosity (LOH) and may precondition a cell towards tumorigenecity, while still appearing histologically normal.[19] In addition, epigenetic modification of the genome, such as promoter methylation, is another mechanism of genomic instability that can further contribute to head and neck carcinogenesis.[20] The overall result of these molecular alterations leads to aberrant protein expression and function, which impacts cellular processes that regulate DNA repair, apoptosis, cell cycle progression, and proliferation.[21] Taking advantage of techniques that can be used to detect these molecular alterations, we can develop these events as molecular markers to more accurately assess the surgical margins.

Genetic Events in the Head and Neck Squamous Cell Carcinoma Model of Progression as Molecular Surgical Markers

In an attempt to model the progression of HNSCC, Califano and colleagues[16] used polymerase chain reaction (PCR)-based microsatellite analysis to evaluate genetic alterations, specifically LOH, in microscopic lesions at varying histopathological stages. Tissues histopathologically presented as

Table 1
Proposal for revised classification of secondary cancers after the removal of a primary head and neck squamous cell carcinoma

Histopathological Assessment	
Second tumor:	
Distance <2 cm; <3 y between diagnoses	Local recurrence
Distance >2 cm; >3 y between diagnoses	Second primary tumor
Molecular Assessment	
Second tumor:	
Identical molecular pattern; proximity to first primary tumor	Local recurrence
Similar molecular pattern; defected field of first primary tumor	Second field tumor
Distinct molecular pattern; distal to first primary tumor	Second primary tumor

Histopathological assessment is based on the previous criteria of proximity and time between diagnoses. Molecular assessment incorporates genetic information to understand the association between first and secondary tumors.

normal, different severity of dysplasia (premalignant), and malignant, contain a pattern of "early" and "late" genomic events that contribute to the development of HNSCC (**Fig. 1**). These genetic events, which can occur in normal-appearing tissues adjacent to the gross tumors, are reflective of the theory of field cancerization and may be used as molecular markers of premalignancy to more accurately assess the surgical margin of HNSCC.

This progression model revealed LOH involving 9p21 to 22 as an early event in HNSCC, as it was observed in epithelial hyperplastic lesions. Retrospective examination of histopathologically tumor-free surgical margins indicated that LOH at 9p21 in the adjacent tissues of HNSCC resected tumors was prognostic for an increased local recurrence for patients, with a hazard ratio of 3.167.[22] Approximately 70% of HNSCC tumors display an alteration in this chromosomal region,[23] and additional studies have revealed this chromosomal region to be associated the *CDKN2A* gene, which encodes the tumor suppressor protein p16.[24,25] p16 is an important cell cycle regulator and has been shown to be frequently inactivated in HNSCC via homozygous deletion (67%) and increased methylation of its respective promotor (21%), resulting in decreased p16 protein expression.[25] When researchers paired PCR and Western blot analysis to investigate the molecular characteristics of p16 in HNSCC, only 19% of the tumors displayed mutated p16, whereas p16 protein expression was reduced in 69% of the tumors.[26] This latter study did not observe p16

mutations in normal or premalignant tissues, but did observe reduced expression of the p16 protein. This suggests that the use of p16 protein expression or gene methylation patterns may be more accurate in assessing the surgical margin in HNSCC, rather than mutations in the p16 gene.

Subsequent genetic events observed in the HNSCC model involved the loci 3p and 17p, which were observed in histopathologically classified dysplastic lesions. LOH of 3p has been reported at rates up to 67%.[27] Genes associated with 3p include *FHIT* and *RASSF1A*; however, their potential functional roles in HNSCC tumorigenesis have yet to be fully understood.[19] The chromosome region 17p13 is associated with p53 tumor suppressor, which is well-known to be dysregulated in human malignancies of all types,[28] with approximately 50% of HNSCC tumors displaying mutations.[29] One of the earliest studies incorporating assessing mutant *p53* gene in surgical margins of patients with HNSCC was reported by Brennan and colleagues,[30] wherein they sought to detect mutations of p53 gene in surgical margins of the resected HNSCC tumor specimens. Taking advantage of the sensitivity of PCR, the researchers examined histopathologically defined negative margins for specific *p53* mutations identified in the corresponding tumors, and observed no recurrence in the 12 patients who displayed a negative MSM. In contrast, 5 of 13 patients who displayed a positive MSM developed recurrences within 7 months postsurgery. This result prompted van Houten and colleagues,[31] to examine the value of *p53* mutations as a marker for local recurrence in

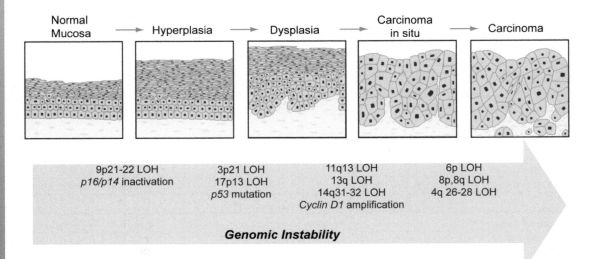

Fig. 1. Genetic model of HNSCC. Phenotypic progression of normal mucosa into carcinoma resulting from an accumulation of genetic alterations. Molecular analysis revealed LOH events, impacting gene expression, facilitate head and neck carcinogenesis.

patients with HNSCC in a larger cohort. Among 76 patients entered into the study, 50 displayed a positive MSM. Of those, 9 patients developed local recurrence and 4 developed regional recurrence. Of note, for those displaying a negative MSM, only 1 patient developed a regional recurrence (no local recurrence was observed).

The progression model showed later genetic events at chromosome regions 11q13, 13q, and 14q31 to 32 that were associated with carcinoma in situ. The Cyclin D1 gene is located at 11q13 region, with approximately 30% of HNSCC tumors displaying amplification of this gene, which can promote cell proliferation.[32,33] This observation prompted the analysis of Cyclin D1 protein overexpression via immunohistochemistry in a cohort of patients.[34] Of 116 patients, 65.6% of the HNSCC tumors displayed Cyclin D1–positive staining, with 45.6% of the patients displaying Cyclin D1–positive surgical margins that were histopathologically defined as tumor-free. When assessing genomic events associated with 13q, patients with laryngeal carcinomas were examined for LOH in 3 regions in the chromosome arm of 13q.[35] Tumor tissues displayed LOH rates ranging from 49% to 64% in the 3 regions, with a higher rate of LOH observed at 13q14 locus, which harbors tumor suppressor gene *RB1*. Further analysis of this same locus revealed an LOH rate of 31% in the negative surgical margins. In HNSCC, approximately 50% of cases display LOH events in 13q,[27] which harbors both tumor suppressor gene *BRCA2* (13q13.1) and *RB1* (13q14.2), as well as the putative suppressor gene *BRCAx* (13q21.2–22.1).[36] Previous studies suggested that RB1 mRNA and protein levels were not significantly altered in HNSCC tumors,[37] suggesting the involvement of other two suppressor genes (1 proximal and 2 distal to *RB1*) with the proximity of the *BRCA* variants in the 13q locus supporting this notion. Further studies would be needed to verify this observation, reveal the associated subsequent inactivation of these genes in head and neck tumorigenesis, as well as their potential implication in MSM analysis.

Genetic alterations observed in the latter stage of the progression model of HNSCC, which involves histopathologically invasive tumors, included LOH events at 6p, 8q, 8p, and 4q26 to 28 chromosome loci. *HLA-1* located on locus 6p is downregulated in HNSCC and associated with LOH at 6p21.3.[38] By downregulating HLA-1, tumor cells can escape detection by the immune system through evading T-cell recognition.[39] Additional genes (loci) associated with a malignant phenotype include *MYC* (8q24.12), *PRKDC* (8q11), and *FGFR1* (8p21), as well as loss of IL2 (4q26).[40] In the latter study, Worsham and colleagues[40] revealed a total of

16 genes, with genomic alterations involving copy loss or gain, which could be used to discriminate between cancer and noncancer tissues. It would be of interest to evaluate the potential application of this gene panel for discriminating premalignant lesions from nontumor tissue and determine if the gene copy pattern displays any predictive value when assessing surgical margins.

In outlining the progression model of HNSCC, we not only obtain a greater understanding of head and neck tumorigenesis, but also identify the associated genomic events. There has been considerable effort to exploit these genetic alterations as molecular markers of head and neck premalignancies that would otherwise go undetected via histopathological examination. Several retrospective studies have shown the utility of these molecular markers to more accurately define surgical margins, and indicated molecular assessment as a stronger prognostic indicator of disease recurrence than morphologic analysis alone.

Methylation Patterns as a Molecular Surgical Margin Marker

Alterations in the patterns of DNA methylation are another common event in developing neoplasia, resulting in gene expression silencing and genomic instability.[41] Hypermethylation of gene promoters results in loss of gene function, and is often associated with tumor suppressor genes that would normally inhibit cancer initiation and progression. In HNSCC, changes in promoter methylation status may not only reveal as a second mechanism of head and neck tumorigenesis, but also may be used as molecular targets in defining status of surgical margins.

One tumor suppressor gene frequently inactivated in HNSCC is p16, an important regulator of the cell cycle.[25] Although this initial study suggested mutations are the common event to inactivate p16, further studies demonstrated that p16 promoter hypermethylation is one of the main causes for p16 loss of function.[42] When researchers compared the methylation patterns of both cancer tissue and adjacent normal-appearing mucosa, they observed p16 promoter methylation in 72% and 27% of the tissues, respectively.[43] These results indicate that hypermethylation of the p16 promoter occurs in histologically "normal" premalignant tissues. When assessing p16 promoter methylation in carcinomas of the tongue, Sinha and colleagues[44] showed that of 38 patients, 86.8% of tumors displayed p16 promoter methylation. When the surgical margins were analyzed, of the 30 patients who displayed histopathologically negative margins,

43.3% displayed positive margins for methylation of the p16 promoter, with a 6.3-fold increased risk of local recurrence relative to those with molecular negative margins. Other studies have examined the utility of p16 promoter methylation as a molecular marker in combination with methylation in other gene promoters, such as MGMT and DAP-K, indicating they can be used to improve sensitivity and more accurately define histopathologically negative surgical margins.[43,45,46] It was found that 64% of patients with HNSCC displayed an informative methylation pattern, when p16 promoter methylation was combined with the methylation patterns of the gene promoters of Cyclin A1 (CCNA1) and DCC Netrin 1 receptor (DCC).[47] When incorporating the methylation information into the MSM analysis of these patients, those with a molecularly negative margin did not display any disease-specific events (ie, local recurrence or metastasis) even 2 years after resection. Interestingly, of 11 patients who displayed a molecularly positive surgical margin, 7 were treated with adjuvant radiotherapy with 1 patient subsequently developing local recurrence, whereas all 4 patients without the follow-up treatment developed disease-specific recurrences. These results suggest MSM assessment also can be used as a criterion for introducing adjuvant therapy postresection, which may further reduce disease recurrence. However, one study showed that when p16 promoter methylation was combined with the methylation patterns of additional gene promoters, including Cytoglobin, E-cadherin, and TMEFF2, these biomarkers failed to provide a prognostic value for the disease recurrence.[48] The conflicting results suggest the importance of selecting the correct promoter targets to evaluate, as not all alterations of promoter methylation contribute equally in terms of their biological roles in HNSCC. Other studies focusing on promoter methylation patterns have revealed additional potential targets that can be used in evaluating the MSM in HNSCC. The mitotic checkpoint gene, CHFR, has been shown to have aberrant promoter methylation in a variety of cancers, with approximately 30% of HNSCC displaying hypermethylation of CHFR promoter.[49] On further investigation in oral squamous cell carcinoma (OSCC), hypermethylation rates were found in up to 46.1%, with 7.7% displaying aberrant CHFR promoter methylation in the adjacent normal-appearing mucosa.[50] Although the investigators did not focus on assessing CHFR promoter hypermethylation in the context of surgical margins or disease recurrence, it would be of interest to examine its potential as a marker in the future. In another study, Hayashi and colleagues[51] performed a prospective study investigating the utility of 6 genes for their predicting value of local recurrence in a small cohort of patients with HNSCC. The investigators identified a 2-gene combination of EDRNA and HOXA9 wherein a positive methylation status of their respective promoters in the surgical margins could be predictive of an increased local recurrence and a reduced overall survival.

There have been extensive studies examining promoter methylation patterns in HNSCC, revealing a variety of tumor suppressor genes and other cell regulatory genes displaying aberrant promoter methylation.[20] However, few assessed the methylation patterns of adjacent normal-appearing mucosa, instead focusing on differences of the promoter methylation difference between the cancer tissues and normal tissue. Although these studies contribute to our understanding of head and neck tumorigenesis and provide an array of potential biomarker targets for HNSCC diagnosis, additional research is needed to establish whether there are individual or panels of novel methylated promoter targets that can be used to assess the MSM. Therefore, further studies with various patient populations and larger cohorts will be necessary to validate the predicting values and proper panel of biomarkers.

Protein Expression as a Molecular Marker in Molecular Surgical Margin Analysis

The HNSCC progression model indicates there are a multitude of genetic events that occur during head and neck tumorigenesis. The genetic alterations can impact cell signaling pathways that would normally regulate cellular activities. As a result of this dysregulation, RNAs and proteins are abnormally expressed, which provides additional molecular marker targets that can be evaluated for their value in accurately defining MSM.

In addition to mutations in the p53 gene, p53 protein expression also can be used as a molecular marker in HNSCC MSM analysis. Mutations in p53 can result in a mutant p53 protein that has an increased half-life, leading to accumulation of the protein in both nuclei and cytoplasm of the cells.[52] Using immunohistochemistry, several studies have revealed overexpression of p53 in 50% to 60% of HNSCC tumors,[53–55] with strong correlation between p53 mutations and the p53 protein overexpression.[56] When assessing p53 immunostaining in 43 patients with OSCC, 27 (62.7%) of the tumors displayed positive p53 staining in cancer tissues; of these, 21 patients displayed positive p53 staining in the nonmalignant adjacent mucosa.[57] Interestingly, of the 16 patients displaying negative p53 staining in the

OSCC tissues, 12 displayed positive p53 staining in the corresponding nonmalignant adjacent mucosa. The investigators noted that one novel aspect of their respective study was assessing the localization of positive p53 staining, wherein they observed the trend of basal p53 staining in the adjacent mucosa was associated with negative p53 staining in the tumors, whereas suprabasal p53 staining of the adjacent mucosa was associated with positive p53 staining in the tumors, suggesting that suprabasal p53 staining in premalignant lesions may be more valuable in predicting local tumor recurrence. In another study, 20 patients with OSCC were examined for both p53 immunoreactivity and in situ hybridization in histopathologically negative resection margins. The investigators observed positive p53 staining in margins of 7 of the patients and chromosomal aneuploidy in margins of 4 additional patients.[58] In the follow-up study, wherein this same patient population was reevaluated for disease recurrence, those who had local recurrence displayed positive MSM involving chromosomal aneuploidy, wherein positive p53 staining in the resection margins was observed in only 3 of the patients.[59] These results prompted the investigators to suggest that chromosomal aneuploidy is more indicative of disease recurrence than positive p53 staining, but conceded that this observation would require additional analysis.

The protein eukaryotic translation initiation factor 4E (eIF4E) was shown to be overexpressed in HNSCC and in some premalignant lesions.[60] To assess the potential utility of eIF4E as an MSM, Nathan and colleagues[61] analyzed eIF4E protein expression in histologically tumor-free surgical margins and its impact on local recurrence. In total, 36 (55%) of 65 patients displayed a positive MSM for the marker eIF4E in histopathologically negative margins, with 56% developing local recurrence. For those patients displaying a negative MSM, only 6.9% developed recurrence, providing evidence for the utility of this protein marker in MSM analysis. However, a recent study investigated both p53 and eIF4E protein expression in histopathologically negative surgical margins and found overexpression of p53 and eIF4E in 54% and 88%, respectively.[62] Although 86% of patients with local recurrence displayed positive eIF4E margins compared with 43% of patients who displayed positive p53 margins (all of whom displayed positive eIF4E margins), no significant association of marker expression and disease recurrence was observed. Similarly, neither eIF4E (83%) nor p53 (53%) expression in the surgical margin was significantly associated with patient mortality. Despite the promising early data, the lack of significance with regard to marker association with disease recurrence and overall survival in the latter study, although comprised of a small sample size, casts doubt of utility of these 2 protein biomarkers in MSM assessment.

Dysregulation of apoptosis is another mechanism cancer cells use for survival. Survivin is an antiapoptotic protein that has been found to be overexpressed in a variety of cancers,[63] and was found to be a prognostic indicator of an invasive and aggressive phenotype in oral cancer.[64] To assess the value of using Survivin to assess MSM in laryngeal cancer, researchers examined 112 cases and found expression of Survivin in 68% of tumors and 39% of histopathologically negative surgical margins.[65] Fifty-nine percent of patients with Survivin-positive surgical margins developed local recurrence compared with only 22% of the patients with Survivin-negative margins. When Survivin staining was paired with staining for the cell adhesion molecule, CD44v6, recurrence incidence rate of 83% compared with 11% (positive vs negative margins) was observed, suggesting the paired-protein MSM analysis has a promising value in predicting the disease recurrence. Although this study focused on only one anatomic site in head and neck, additional studies that evaluate the potential of using Survivin and CD44v6 to assess the MSM in HNSCC would provide further evidence for using these protein markers in the clinical setting.

Proteomic-based technologies have been used in several studies in an attempt to elucidate novel protein biomarkers that could be utilized for diagnostic and prognostic information in HNSCC.[66] In an effort to identify proteins that could be used to detect precursor lesions and predict local recurrence, Schaaij-Visser and colleagues[67] used differential proteomic analysis to reveal candidate biomarker proteins that could distinguish among genetically normal, premalignant, and tumor tissues. The preliminary proteomic analysis revealed 40 differentially expressed proteins, with most expression differences observed between normal mucosa and tumor tissues. To validate candidate biomarker proteins, the investigators used immunohistochemistry staining to retrospectively analyze patients for disease relapse and found that low expression of the proteins keratin-4 and cornulin had a significantly high association with local recurrence. Although the patient sample size used for this study was small, the results clearly illustrate the potential benefit of proteomic analysis to identify novel proteins to be used in evaluating MSM.

As indicated by several studies, protein expression patterns are another method to evaluate MSM in patients with HNSCC. Genetic alterations can result in aberrant protein expression, and due to the functional role of proteins, atypical protein expression can impact a wide range of cellular pathways and further contribute to HNSCC progression. Identifying proteins that are differentially expressed as a result of these genetic events and altered pathways enables their utilization as targets in assessing MSM.

FACTORS TO CONSIDER WHEN SELECTING MARGINS FOR ANALYSIS

When examining the surgical margin, there are several additional aspects that must be considered for an accurate assessment, including defining an adequate margin width, the timing at which the margin analysis is performed, and the manner in which the margin is obtained. Routinely, a surgeon will resect the gross tumor and surrounding area, using ink staining to designate the edge of the resection. During histopathological evaluation, the distance of tumor or atypical tissue relative to the inked edge is evaluated to determine if the surgical margin is adequate. As noted by Hinni and colleagues,[68] an arbitrary definition of ≥5 mm has been considered an adequate surgical margin, but studies have reported a wide range of margins (2 mm to 10 mm) with varying corresponding rates of locoregional recurrence and overall survival. Further investigation in a large cohort of patients with oral cancer revealed a similar recurrence rate (approximately 25%) and 5-year survival (approximately 70%) between margins greater than 3 mm and greater than 5 mm, indicating that the arbitrary surgical margin of ≥5 mm being considered adequate may require revision.[69] As previously discussed, there are a variety of genetic, epigenetic, and protein expression alterations in histopathologically normal-appearing cells that could serve as molecular markers indicative of premalignant conditions. Of interest would be to evaluate the proximity of positive molecular markers relative to the inked edge. Not only could these markers be used to differentiate between positive and negative MSMs, but also be evaluated to better define the adequate width between the inked resection edge and the defected field.

An important aspect of examining the surgical margin is the speed at which a test report can be generated and returned to the surgeon regarding the margin status. Currently, a surgical margin greater than 5 mm is considered adequate.[70] If histopathological analysis reveals a positive surgical margin, re-resection can be performed until a negative margin is achieved, with a similar rate of local recurrence control observed as initial resections displaying negative margins.[71] However, some anatomic sites limit the extent of this macroscopic margin, which can then significantly impact the histopathological negative status of the surgical margin, while the ability to perform repeat resection may be limited due to the necessity of immediate reconstructive surgery. Intraoperative frozen-section evaluation (FSE) of surgical margins has been used in HNSCC in an effort to provide rapid pathologic assessment regarding margin status before surgery closure and reconstruction.[72] Regular histopathology of the margins is then performed. FSE has shown a similar concordance as the processed sections in some studies.[73] However, the overall utility of intraoperative FSE has also been questioned, with reported accuracy rate of evaluating close or positive margins at approximately 71.3%.[74] This lower rate of accuracy has been attributed to several factors, including the site from which the specimen is obtained, sampling error, and tissue shrinkage.[75–77] Inclusion of molecular characteristics for intraoperative margin assessment may increase the specificity and sensitivity of surgical margin assessment. To test the feasibility of this approach, Goldenberg and colleagues[45] used quantitative methylation-specific PCR (QMSP) to determine the hypermethylation pattern of p16 and MGMT promoters in the surgical margins. Although the number of patients was small in the study, the investigators showed that QMSP analysis could be performed within a period conducive to intraoperative assessment. Other studies are needed to verify this protocol, but these preliminary results illustrate the potential utility of molecular assessment of the surgical margin intraoperatively.

One of the major factors that can significantly impact accurate assessment of the surgical margins is how the margins themselves are obtained (**Fig. 2**). During surgery, a surgeon can obtain margins that are parallel to the plane of the resection (en face) via cavity shaving, or right angle to the plane of the resection (perpendicular).[78,79] The benefit of en face margin assessment is that this technique allows for a larger area of the lesion and surrounding tissue to be assessed. In addition, when taken from the mucosal edge, en face margins can be a much more definitive assessment of whether residual tumor remains. However, some disadvantages of en face margin assessment include difficulty for the pathologist ascertaining the width of the tumor margin, as well as determining tumor involvement in deep connecting tissues. Perpendicular margins, which involve removing a tissue section from the resection

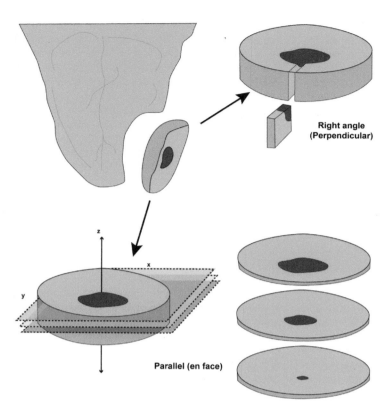

Fig. 2. Contrasting methods to obtain resection sample for surgical margin analysis. Right angle (perpendicular) margin versus parallel (en face) margin obtain via cavity shaving.

Right angle (Perpendicular)

Parallel (en face)

edge to invasive tumor front, facilitate the margin width to be assessed. However, perpendicular margins examine only a small area of the resected tissue, limiting the extent of examination, which can result in false-negative assessments. To overcome this, a pathologist may assess multiple sections in the resected tissue, removing slices from the surface into deeper regions of the sample; however, even supplementary sections may still result in an inaccurate marginal assessment. If the resected samples were to contain sufficient material, the best approach in assessing the margin would be combining both en face and perpendicular examination of the resected tissue, which would combine the advantages of each technique and reduce inherent biases.

LIMITATIONS OF MOLECULAR SURGICAL MARGINS

Incorporating molecular markers to accurately assess the surgical margin in HNSCC has shown a great deal of promise; however, there are several aspects that warrant further discussion that may limit their utility in the clinical setting. In reviewing the literature and discussing the multitude of molecular markers that have been evaluated for use

in the MSM, one factor that limits their application is the respective low coverage of these markers within the surgical margin. As an example, the use of mutant p53 as an MSM is limited by the number of patients displaying this alteration, as Poeta and colleagues[80] reported only 50% of HNSCC tumors harbor a mutation in p53. Further confounding the use of p53 in the MSM is that in this same study, the investigators categorized the mutations in p53 as "nondisruptive" and "disruptive," revealing heterogeneity of p53 mutations that vary with regard to impact on overall survival. The low coverage, myriad of mutations, and ability to stratify those mutations that impair biological function make it difficult to develop simple assays that can be integrated into the clinical setting, and limit the utility of mutant p53. Other examples, which include the early genetic event involving LOH at 9p21 to 22, observed in approximately 70% of HNSCC cases, dysregulation of p16, either via homozygous deletion (67%) or increased promoter methylation (21%), or p53 protein expression (50%–60%) illustrate that no marker is expressed homogeneously.

Another aspect that limits the incorporation of the MSM into the clinical setting is the amount of time needed to perform these molecular analyses.

Intraoperative examination facilitates real-time assessment of the surgical margin that allows the surgeon to determine whether a negative margin has been obtained, or if additional resection is necessary. Unlike histopathological assessment via FSE, the time needed to detect molecular alterations may preclude their intraoperative utility. However, the development of methodologies and advances in instrumentation have enabled rapid assessment of the surgical margin using p53 mutations,[81] promoter methylation patterns,[45] and protein expression.[61] As more studies examining the MSM in HNSCC integrate intraoperative time constraints into their experimental design, the feasibility of using MSM in the clinical setting will become more realistic.

Possibly the most significant concern that arises regarding the use of molecular alterations for assessing the surgical margin is determining a particular biomarker's predictive value with regard to malignant disease. It has been shown that LOH at 9p21 and 3p are early genetic events in HNSCC, with approximately 51% of premalignant lesions displaying altered genetic events at either or both loci.[82] However, within this patient population, only 37% developed HNSCC. These results raise the important question of how to approach surgical resection when histopathologically normal tissues display genetic alterations that may not necessarily develop into malignancy. In addition, clinicians must consider incidences of false-positive results that may arise due to detecting a molecular marker that may be derived from another source. It has been shown that mutant DNA fragments can been detected in saliva, indicating that tumor DNA is released by cancerous cells into the proximal area.[83] With the sensitivity of current DNA sequencing technology, the inability to sample the entire resection surface may result in false-positives resulting from mutant DNA detected in the surgical margin that may come from secondary sources (ie, gross tumor). Other molecular targets or methodologies may preclude these issues of specificity and sensitivity, but whereas histopathology may include biases toward interpretation and subjectivity, the MSM includes distinct factors that must be acknowledged and addressed as well.

EMERGING RESEARCH AND FUTURE DIRECTIONS

In the past few years, there have been rapid advances in technology that have not only expanded our understanding of head and neck carcinogenesis, but also have facilitated the development of novel strategies that may be incorporated into the treatment of HNSCC. Several studies have incorporated next generation sequencing (NGS) in an attempt to elucidate the mutational landscape associated with HNSCC.[84–86] These studies revealed a myriad of gene mutations and their frequency in HNSCC, including those previously known such as p53 (30%–72%) and CDKN2A (12%–22%), as well as novel genes including NOTCH1 (8%–19%). Further investigation into NOTCH1 revealed many of the mutations resulted in truncated gene product, which would lead to inactivation of the protein and indicated that NOTCH1 may function as a tumor suppressor in HNSCC.[87] However, additional investigation into NOTCH signaling has contradicted this hypothesis, wherein a subset of tumors showed increased expression of NOTCH1 independent of the mutation status, indicating a bimodal function of NOTCH1 in HNSCC.[88]

One of the more interesting observations from these NGS studies involves the delineation of distinct gene profiles relating to 2 subtypes of HNSCC. Heavy smoking and alcohol consumption are well-known risk factors for HNSCC, but recently the human papillomavirus (HPV) has been shown to be a significant risk factor in HNSCC,[89] accounting for almost 25% of head and neck cancer cases.[90] Not only do HPV-negative and HPV-positive tumors display differing prognosis and disease recurrence patterns, but also distinct mutation patterns: HPV-negative tumors display a twofold increase in mutations relative to HPV-positive tumors.[84] Specifically, mutations in tumor suppressor genes, such as p53 and the putative tumor suppressor gene NOTCH1 are observed more frequently in HPV-negative tumors, whereas mutations in the oncogene PIK3CA are associated with HPV-positive tumors.[86] This observation has implications for the development of precision therapies, as activation mutations in signaling proteins may be targeted, whereas inactivating mutations are not "druggable" and surgical intervention is the best course of treatment. Overall, these results illustrate the heterogeneity of HNSCC, and that various subtypes, derived from distinct etiologic sources, can be categorized by their unique mutation signature that influences, and potentially limits, treatment options.

Improvements in mass spectrometry instrumentation and methods have expanded the utility of this technology in HNSCC tissue analysis. Exploratory mass spectrometry–based proteomic studies have attempted to identify novel protein targets that may be used to distinguish genetically altered mucosa that are histologically normal.[67,91,92] In addition, the ability of mass spectrometry instruments to detect a wide a variety of compounds has facilitated the development of mass spectrometry imaging, wherein the spatial distribution of biological molecules can be visualized by their molecular masses, and has been applied to assess surgical margin in a variety of cancers.[93–95] Rapid evaporative ionization mass spectrometry (REIMS) is an exciting technology that enables real-time analysis of aerosols generated during electrosurgical dissection.[96] When this technique was coupled to the iKnife, a specialized electrosurgical device, real-time analysis of in vivo tissue facilitated intraoperative assessment of the surgical margin in a variety of cancers with greater than 95% sensitivity and specificity.[97] Current limitations of the REIMS technique include the requirement of a spectral database to be generated before intraoperative assessment, as well as biasness toward detecting lipid-based molecules, which ionize more readily. As ionization methodologies are improved to include a broad array of biological molecules, and the number of spectral libraries increases, REIMS may prove to be one of the most flexible techniques for intraoperative assessment of the MSM.

REFERENCES

1. American Cancer Society. Cancer facts & figures 2015. American Cancer Society; 2015. http://dx.doi.org/10.3322/caac.21254.
2. Haque R, Contreras R, McNicoll MP, et al. Surgical margins and survival after head and neck cancer surgery. BMC Ear Nose Throat Disord 2006;6:2.
3. Varvares MA, Poti S, Kenyon B, et al. Surgical margins and primary site resection in achieving local control in oral cancer resections. Laryngoscope 2015;125(10):2298–307.
4. Upile T, Fisher C, Jerjes W, et al. The uncertainty of the surgical margin in the treatment of head and neck cancer. Oral Oncol 2007;43(4):321–6.
5. Meier JD, Oliver DA, Varvares MA. Surgical margin determination in head and neck oncology: current clinical practice. The results of an International American Head and Neck Society Member Survey. Head Neck 2005;27(11):952–8.
6. Perez-Ordonez B. Molecular biology of squamous cell carcinoma of the head and neck. J Clin Pathol 2006;59(5):445–53.
7. Westra W, Sidransky D. Phenotypic and genotypic disparity in premalignant lesions: of calm water and crocodiles. J Natl Cancer Inst 1998;90(20):1500–1.
8. Mao L, El-Naggar AK, Papadimitrakopoulou V, et al. Phenotype and genotype of advanced premalignant head and neck lesions after chemopreventive therapy. J Natl Cancer Inst 1998;90(20):1545–51.
9. Leemans CR, Tiwari R, Nauta JJP, et al. Recurrence at the primary site in head and neck-cancer and the significance of neck lymph-node metastases as a prognostic factor. Cancer 1994;73(1):187–90.
10. de Carvalho AC, Kowalski LP, Campos AHJFM, et al. Clinical significance of molecular alterations in histologically negative surgical margins of head and neck cancer patients. Oral Oncol 2012;48(3):240–8.
11. Warren S, Gates O. Multiple primary malignant tumors: a survey of the literature and a statistical study. Am J Cancer 1932;16:1358–414.
12. Braakhuis BJM, Tabor MP, René Leemans C, et al. Second primary tumors and field cancerization in oral and oropharyngeal cancer: molecular techniques provide new insights and definitions. Head Neck 2002;24(2):198–206.
13. Slaughter DP, Southwick HW, Smejkal W. Field cancerization in oral stratified squamous epithelium; clinical implications of multicentric origin. Cancer 1953;6(5):963–8.
14. Braakhuis BJM, Bloemena E, Leemans CR, et al. Molecular analysis of surgical margins in head and neck cancer: more than a marginal issue. Oral Oncol 2010;46(7):485–91.
15. Fearon ER, Vogeistein B. A genetic model for colorectal tumorigenesis. Cell 1990;61(5):759–67.
16. Califano J, van der Riet P, Westra W, et al. Genetic progression model for head and neck cancer: implications for field cancerization. Cancer Res 1996;56(11):2488–92.
17. Tabor MP, Brakenhoff RH, Ruijter-Schippers HJ, et al. Multiple head and neck tumors frequently originate from a single preneoplastic lesion. Am J Pathol 2002;161(3):1051–60.
18. Hanahan D, Weinberg RA. Hallmarks of cancer. Cell 2000;100(1):57–70. Available at: http://www.ncbi.nlm.nih.gov/pubmed/10647931.
19. Kim MM, Califano JA. Molecular pathology of head-and-neck cancer. Int J Cancer 2004;112(4):545–53.
20. Demokan S, Dalay N. Role of DNA methylation in head and neck cancer. Clin Epigenetics 2011;2:123–50.
21. Scully C, Field JK, Tanzawa H. Genetic aberrations in oral or head and neck squamous cell carcinoma (SCCHN): 1. Carcinogen metabolism, DNA repair and cell cycle control. Oral Oncol 2000;36(3):256–63.
22. Graveland AP, Golusinski PJ, Buijze M, et al. Loss of heterozygosity at 9p and p53 immunopositivity in surgical margins predict local relapse in head and neck squamous cell carcinoma. Int J Cancer 2011;128(8):1852–9.
23. van der Riet P, Nawroz H, Hruban RH, et al. Frequent loss of chromosome 9p21-22 early in head and neck cancer progression. Cancer Res 1994;54(5):1156–8.
24. Kamb A, Gruis NA, Weaver-Feldhaus J, et al. A cell cycle regulator potentially involved in genesis of many tumor types. Science 1994;264(5157):436–40.

25. Reed AL, Califano J, Cairns P, et al. High frequency of p16 (CDKN2/MTS-1/INK4A) inactivation in head and neck squamous cell carcinoma. Cancer Res 1996;56(16):3630–3. Available at: http://cancerres.aacrjournals.org/content/56/16/3630.short.

26. Sartor M, Steingrimsdottir H, Elamin F, et al. Role of p16/MTS1, cyclin D1 and RB in primary oral cancer and oral cancer cell lines. Br J Cancer 1999;80(1–2): 79–86.

27. Nawroz H, van der Riet P, Hruban RH, et al. Allelotype of head and neck squamous cell carcinoma. Cancer Res 1994;54:1152–5.

28. Hollstein M, Sidransky D, Vogelstein B, et al. p53 mutations in human cancers. Science 1991; 253(5015):49–53.

29. Boyle JO, Hakim J, Koch W, et al. The incidence of p53 mutations increases with progression of head and neck cancer. Cancer Res 1993;53(19): 4477–80.

30. Brennan JA, Mao L, Hruban RH, et al. Molecular assessment of histopathological staging in squamous-cell carcinoma of the head and neck. N Engl J Med 1995;332(7):429–35.

31. van Houten VMM, Leemans CR, Kummer JA, et al. Molecular diagnosis of surgical margins and local recurrence in head and neck cancer patients: a prospective study. Clin Cancer Res 2004;10(11): 3614–20.

32. Callender T, El-Naggar AK, Lee MS, et al. PRAD-1 (CCND1)/cyclin D1 oncogene amplification in primary head and neck squamous cell carcinoma. Cancer 1994;74(1):152–8.

33. Jares P, Fernandez PL, Campo E, et al. PRAD-1/cyclin D1 gene amplification correlates with messenger RNA overexpression and tumor progression in human laryngeal carcinomas. Cancer Res 1994;54(17):4813–7. Available at: http://www.ncbi.nlm.nih.gov/entrez/query.fcgi?cmd=Retrieve&db=PubMed&dopt=Citation&list_uids=8062283.

34. Sakashita T, Homma A, Suzuki S, et al. Prognostic value of cyclin D1 expression in tumor-free surgical margins in head and neck squamous cell carcinomas. Acta Otolaryngol 2013;133(9):984–91.

35. Szukała K, Brieger J, Bruch K, et al. Loss of heterozygosity on chromosome arm 13q in larynx cancer patients: analysis of tumor, margin and clinically unchanged mucosa. Med Sci Monit 2004;10(6): 233–41.

36. Sabbir MG, Roy A, Mandal S, et al. Deletion mapping of chromosome 13q in head and neck squamous cell carcinoma in Indian patients: correlation with prognosis of the tumour. Int J Exp Pathol 2006;87(2):151–61.

37. Maestro R, Piccinin S, Doglioni C, et al. Chromosome 13q deletion mapping in head and neck squamous cell carcinomas: identification of two distinct regions of preferential loss. Cancer Res 1996;56(5):1146–50. Available at: http://www.ncbi.nlm.nih.gov/pubmed/8640775.

38. Feenstra M, Veltkamp M, van Kuik J, et al. HLA class I expression and chromosomal deletions at 6p and 15q in head and neck squamous cell carcinomas. Tissue Antigens 1999;54(3):235–45.

39. Ferris RL. Immunology and immunotherapy of head and neck cancer. J Clin Oncol 2015;33(29): 3293–304.

40. Worsham MJ, Lu M, Chen KM, et al. Malignant and nonmalignant gene signatures in squamous head and neck cancer. J Oncol 2012;2012:1–8.

41. Jones PA, Baylin SB. The fundamental role of epigenetic events in cancer. Nat Rev Genet 2002;3(6): 415–28.

42. El-naggar AK, Lai S, Clayman G, et al. Methylation, a major mechanism of p16/CDKN2 gene inactivation in head and neck squamous carcinoma. Am J Pathol 1997;151(6):1767–74.

43. Kato K, Hara A, Kuno T, et al. Aberrant promoter hypermethylation of p16 and MGMT genes in oral squamous cell carcinomas and the surrounding normal mucosa. J Cancer Res Clin Oncol 2006; 132:735–43.

44. Sinha P, Bahadur S, Thakar A, et al. Significance of promoter hypermethylation of p16 gene for margin assessment in carcinoma tongue. Head Neck 2009;31:1423–30.

45. Goldenberg D, Harden S, Masayesva BG, et al. Intraoperative molecular margin analysis in head and neck cancer. Arch Otolaryngol Head Neck Surg 2004;130(1):39–44.

46. Martone T, Gillio-Tos A, De Marco L, et al. Association between hypermethylated tumor and paired surgical margins in head and neck squamous cell carcinomas. Clin Cancer Res 2007;13(17): 5089–94.

47. Tan HK, Saulnier P, Auperin A, et al. Quantitative methylation analyses of resection margins predict local recurrences and disease-specific deaths in patients with head and neck squamous cell carcinomas. Br J Cancer 2008;99(2):357–63.

48. Shaw RJ, Hobkirk AJ, Nikolaidis G, et al. Molecular staging of surgical margins in oral squamous cell carcinoma using promoter methylation of p16(INK4A), cytoglobin, E-cadherin, and TMEFF2. Ann Surg Oncol 2013;20(8):2796–802.

49. Toyota M, Sasaki Y, Satoh A, et al. Epigenetic inactivation of CHFR in human tumors. Proc Natl Acad Sci U S A 2003;100(13):7818–23.

50. Baba S, Hara A, Kato K, et al. Aberrant promoter hypermethylation of the CHFR gene in oral squamous cell carcinomas. Oncol Rep 2009;22(5):1173–9.

51. Hayashi M, Wu G, Roh J-L, et al. Correlation of gene methylation in surgical margin imprints with locoregional recurrence in head and neck squamous cell carcinoma. Cancer 2015;121(12):1957–65.

52. Bourhis J, Lubin R, Roche B, et al. Analysis of p53 serum antibodies in patients with head and neck squamous cell carcinoma. J Natl Cancer Inst 1996; 88(17):1228–33.

53. Watling DL, Gown AM, Coltrera MD. Overexpression of p53 in head and neck cancer. Head Neck 1992; 14(6):437–44.

54. Field JK, Spandidos DA, Stell PM. Overexpression of p53 gene in head-and-neck cancer, linked with heavy smoking and drinking. Lancet 1992; 339(8791):502–3.

55. Sauter ER, Cleveland D, Trock B, et al. p53 is over-expressed in fifty percent of pre-invasive lesions of head and neck epithelium. Carcinogenesis 1994; 15(10):2269–74.

56. Ahomadegbe JC, Barrois M, Fogel S, et al. High incidence of p53 alterations (mutation, deletion, overexpression) in head and neck primary tumors and metastases; absence of correlation with clinical outcome. Frequent protein overexpression in normal epithelium and in early non-invasive lesions. Onco-gene 1995;10(6):1217–27.

57. Cruz IB, Meijer CJ, Snijders PJ, et al. P53 immunoex-pression in non-malignant oral mucosa adjacent to oral squamous cell carcinoma: potential conse-quences for clinical management. J Pathol 2000; 191(2):132–7.

58. van der Toorn PP, Veltman JA, Bot FJ, et al. Mapping of resection margins of oral cancer for p53 overex-pression and chromosome instability to detect re-sidual (pre)malignant cells. J Pathol 2001;193(1): 66–72.

59. Bergshoeff V, Hopman A, Zwijnenberg I, et al. Chro-mosome instability in resection margins predicts recurrence of oral squamous cell carcinoma. J Pathol 2008;215:347–8.

60. Nathan CAO, Liu L, Li BD, et al. Detection of the proto-oncogene eIF4E in surgical margins may pre-dict recurrence in head and neck cancer. Oncogene 1997;15(5):579–84.

61. Nathan CAO, Franklin S, Abreo FW, et al. Anal-ysis of surgical margins with the molecular marker eIF4E: A prognostic factor in patients with head and neck cancer. J Clin Oncol 1999; 17(9):2909–14.

62. Singh J, Jayaraj R, Baxi S, et al. Immunohistochem-ical expression levels of p53 and eIF4E markers in histologically negative surgical margins, and their association with the clinical outcome of patients with head and neck squamous cell carcinoma. Mol Clin Oncol 2016;4:166–72.

63. Fukuda S, Pelus LM. Survivin, a cancer target with an emerging role in normal adult tissues. Mol Cancer Ther 2006;5(5):1087–98.

64. Lo Muzio L, Farina A, Rubini C, et al. Survivin as prognostic factor in squamous cell carcinoma of the oral cavity. Cancer Lett 2005;225:27–33.

65. Zhao H, Ren J, Zhuo X, et al. Prognostic significance of Survivin and CD44v6 in laryngeal cancer surgical margins. J Cancer Res Clin Oncol 2008;134(10): 1051–8.

66. Schaaij-Visser TBM, Brakenhoff RH, Leemans CR, et al. Protein biomarker discovery for head and neck cancer. J Proteomics 2010;73(10):1790–803.

67. Schaaij-visser TBM, Graveland AP, Gauci S. Differ-ential proteomics identifies protein biomarkers that predict local relapse of head and neck squamous cell carcinomas local relapse of head and neck squamous cell carcinomas. Clin Cancer Res 2009; 15(24):7666–76.

68. Hinni ML, Ferlito A, Brandwein-Gensler MS, et al. Surgical margins in head and neck cancer: a contemporary review. Head Neck 2015;35(9): 1362–70.

69. Nason RW, Binahmed A, Pathak KA, et al. What is the adequate margin of surgical resection in oral cancer? Oral Surg Oral Med Oral Pathol Oral Radiol Endod 2009;107(5):625–9.

70. Lee JA. Standards and datasets for reporting can-cers datasets for histopathology reports on head and neck carcinomas and salivary neoplasms. 2nd edition. London: The Royal College of Pathologists; 2005.

71. Jäckel MC, Ambrosch P, Martin A, et al. Impact of re-resection for inadequate margins on the prognosis of upper aerodigestive tract cancer treated by laser microsurgery. Laryngoscope 2007;117(2):350–6.

72. Black C, Marotti J, Zarovnaya E, et al. Critical evalu-ation of frozen section margins in head and neck cancer resections. Cancer 2006;107(12):2792–800.

73. Ord RA, Aisner S. Accuracy of frozen sections in assessing margins in oral cancer resection. J Oral Maxillofac Surg 1997;55(7):663–9 [discus-sion: 669–71]. Available at: http://www.ncbi.nlm.nih. gov/pubmed/9216496.

74. DiNardo LJ, Lin J, Karageorge LS, et al. Accuracy, utility, and cost of frozen section margins in head and neck cancer surgery. Laryngoscope 2000;110: 1773–6.

75. Cheng A, Cox D, Schmidt BL. Oral squamous cell carcinoma margin discrepancy after resection and pathologic processing. J Oral Maxillofac Surg 2008;66(3):523–9.

76. Olson SM, Hussaini M, Lewis JS. Frozen section analysis of margins for head and neck tumor resec-tions: reduction of sampling errors with a third histo-logic level. Mod Pathol 2011;24(5):665–70.

77. El-Fol HA, Noman SA, Beheiri MG, et al. Significance of post-resection tissue shrinkage on surgical margins of oral squamous cell carcinoma. J Craniomaxillofac Surg 2015;43(4):475–82.

78. Wenig BM. Intraoperative consultation in oral cavity mucosal lesions. In: Atlas of head and neck pathology. Atlas of surgical pathology. 3rd edition.

Amsterdam: Elsevier Health Sciences; 2015. p. 384–96. Available at: https://books.google.com/books?id=wxvYCQAAQBAJ.

79. Demian N. Pitfalls in determining head and neck surgical margins. In: Adjunctive technologies in the management of head and neck pathology. The clinics: surgery. Amsterdam: Elsevier Health Sciences; 2014. p. 151–62. Available at: https://books.google.com/books?id=nyihAwAAQBAJ.

80. Poeta ML, Manola J, Goldwasser MA, et al. TP53 mutations and survival in squamous-cell carcinoma of the head and neck. N Engl J Med 2007;357(25): 2552–61.

81. Harden SV, Thomas DC, Benoit N, et al. Real-time gap ligase chain reaction: a rapid semiquantitative assay for detecting p53 mutation at low levels in surgical margins and lymph nodes from resected lung and head and neck tumors. Clin Cancer Res 2004; 10(7):2379–85.

82. Mao L, Lee JS, Fan YH, et al. Frequent microsatellite alterations at chromosomes 9p21 and 3p14 in oral premalignant lesions and their value in cancer risk assessment. Nat Med 1996;2(6):682–5.

83. Wang YX, Springer S, Mulvey CL, et al. Detection of somatic mutations and HPV in the saliva and plasma of patients with head and neck squamous cell carcinomas. Sci Transl Med 2015;7(293):293ra104.

84. Stransky N, Egloff AM, Tward AD, et al. The mutational landscape of head and neck squamous cell carcinoma. Science 2011;333(6046):1157–60.

85. Gaykalova DA, Mambo E, Choudhary A, et al. Novel insight into mutational landscape of head and neck squamous cell carcinoma. PLoS One 2014;9(3):1–9.

86. Lawrence MS, Sougnez C, Lichtenstein L, et al. Comprehensive genomic characterization of head and neck squamous cell carcinomas. Nature 2015; 517(7536):576–82.

87. Agrawal N, Frederick MJ, Pickering CR, et al. Exome sequencing of head and neck squamous cell carcinoma reveals inactivating mutations in NOTCH1. Science 2011;333(6046):1154–7.

88. Sun W, Gaykalova DA, Ochs MF, et al. Activation of the NOTCH pathway in head and neck cancer. Cancer Res 2014;74(4):1091–104.

89. Kostareli E, Holzinger D, Hess J. New concepts for translational head and neck oncology: lessons from HPV-related oropharyngeal squamous cell carcinomas. Front Oncol 2012;2:1–10.

90. Rizzo G, Black M, Mymryk J, et al. Defining the genomic landscape of head and neck cancers through next-generation sequencing. Oral Dis 2015; 21(1):e11–24.

91. Baker H, Patel V, Molinolo AA, et al. Proteome-wide analysis of head and neck squamous cell carcinomas using laser-capture microdissection and tandem mass spectrometry. Oral Oncol 2005;41(2): 183–99.

92. Roesch-Ely M, Nees M, Karsai S, et al. Proteomic analysis reveals successive aberrations in protein expression from healthy mucosa to invasive head and neck cancer. Oncogene 2007;26(1):54–64.

93. Caldwell RL, Gonzalez A, Oppenheimer SR, et al. Molecular assessment of the tumor protein microenvironment using imaging mass spectrometry. Cancer Genomics Proteomics 2006;3:279–88.

94. Eberlin LS, Tibshirani RJ, Zhang J, et al. Molecular assessment of surgical-resection margins of gastric cancer by mass-spectrometric imaging. Proc Natl Acad Sci U S A 2014;111(7):2436–41.

95. Calligaris D, Caragacianu D, Liu X, et al. Application of desorption electrospray ionization mass spectrometry imaging in breast cancer margin analysis. Proc Natl Acad Sci 2014;111(42):15184–9.

96. Balog J, Szaniszló T, Schaefer KC, et al. Identification of biological tissues by rapid evaporative ionization mass spectrometry. Anal Chem 2010;82(17): 7343–50.

97. Balog J, Sasi-Szabó L, Kinross J, et al. Intraoperative tissue identification using rapid evaporative ionization mass spectrometry. Sci Transl Med 2013; 5(194):194ra93.

Margin Analysis
Squamous Cell Carcinoma of the Oral Cavity

 CrossMark

Michael Shapiro, DDS, MA[a], Andrew Salama, DDS, MD[b],*

KEYWORDS

- Surgical margin • Oral squamous cell carcinoma • Margin shrinkage • Frozen sections

KEY POINTS

- There is a relationship between locoregional control and margin status. A minimum of 5 mm of tumor-free tissue is considered a clear margin.
- The utility of frozen sections in oral squamous cell carcinoma is controversial; however, frozen sections may give the surgeon an additional opportunity to prevent an ultimately positive margin.
- Specimen-driven margins appear to be more predictive of actual margin status than defect-driven margins.
- There is a role for adjuvant chemo-radiotherapy in patients with close or positive margin status.

Oral squamous cell carcinoma (OSCC) is the most common oral malignancy, accounting for more than 90% of oral cancers. In the United States, OSCC represents nearly 4% of all annually diagnosed malignancies, and nearly 32,000 new cases of OSCC are anticipated in 2016, with more than 6000 cancer-related deaths.[1] A primary management principle for most oral cavity cancers is complete surgical excision, and a "negative margin" on final pathology. This article primarily focuses on defining terms, including negative margin, close margin, and positive margin, and, furthermore, delineates the current role of frozen section analysis and adjuvant therapy in treating OSCC with respect to surgical margin status.

Initial assessment of OSCC begins with a thorough clinical evaluation. Of paramount importance is a complete evaluation of all anatomic structures in the oral cavity by both visual examination and palpation. The examination may be aided by the use of pan-endoscopy under anesthesia if the tumor is located in an area that is painful or difficult to evaluate. In addition to a scrupulous evaluation of the oral cavity, a careful examination of the cervical lymph nodes is a vital aspect of the initial assessment of OSCC. Manual palpation, computed tomography (CT) scan and PET/CT scan are routinely used to assess both regional and distant metastases. A fat-suppressed, contrast-enhanced neck MRI is useful in select cases, as it may allow the clinician to view the neck in planes not available by CT. After a comprehensive workup is completed and the patient is staged, the decision to proceed with surgical resection is usually determined by a multidisciplinary group of treating specialists. The prognosis of OSCC is influenced by many factors, including tumor size and stage, depth of invasion, tumor grade, lymphovascular and perineural invasion, extranodal extension, and patient age and distant metastases.[2–5] Although these factors are predetermined and cannot be influenced by the surgeon, the surgeon has the greatest capacity to influence the surgical margin, which is an important independent prognosticator.[6–11]

[a] Department of Oral and Maxillofacial Surgery, Boston Medical Center, 100 East Newton Street, Suite G-407, Boston, MA 02118, USA; [b] Department of Oral and Maxillofacial Surgery, Boston Medical Center, Boston University School of Dental Medicine, 100 East Newton Street, Suite G-407, Boston, MA 02118, USA
* Corresponding author.
E-mail address: Andrew.Salama@bmc.org

Oral Maxillofacial Surg Clin N Am 29 (2017) 259–267
http://dx.doi.org/10.1016/j.coms.2017.03.003
1042-3699/17/© 2017 Elsevier Inc. All rights reserved.

Clear surgical margins are an important prognosticator for local control and disease-specific survival. A recent meta-analysis investigated the relationship between surgical margins and local recurrence in OSCC. A 21% absolute risk reduction in local recurrence was associated with clear surgical margins.[11] The importance of a clear surgical margin and local control was further emphasized in a study by Kurita and colleagues,[7] who found that the 5-year local control rate was 91.0% for a clear margin, 80.4% for a close margin, and just 43.8% for a positive margin.

In the contemporary literature, Looser and colleagues[12] were among the first to opine that a clear surgical margin required a defined distance past the invasive tumor, and suggested a distance of 5 mm. Since then, multiple studies have attempted to elucidate exactly what constitutes a "clear" margin. The most common consensus distance for a clear margin in OSCC is a minimum of 5 mm or more of healthy tissue around the tumor[8–10]; however, some investigators have suggested that 3 mm of surrounding healthy tissue suffices as a clear margin.[13,14] Yamada and colleagues[10] performed a systematic evaluation of the impact of the width of the free margin on surgical outcomes, and found that a tumor with a free margin of 4 mm was associated with an increased risk of local recurrence, whereas a free margin of 5 mm was not associated with a significant risk of local recurrence. This appears to confirm that 5 mm of healthy tissue around the tumor is indeed the minimum acceptable amount for a clear margin.

There is consensus among the Royal college of Pathologists (RCP), the American College of Pathologists (ACP), and the National Comprehensive Cancer Network (NCCN) that to be considered a "negative" margin, the minimal acceptable amount of disease-free tissue is 5 mm. The definition of a "positive" margin is slightly variable, as the ACP defines a positive margin as invasive carcinoma less than 1 mm from the surgical margin, whereas both the RCP and the NCCN define a positive margin as invasive carcinoma or carcinoma-in-situ/high-grade dysplasia present at margins (microscopic cut-through of tumor).

According to the NCCN:

Clear margin: The distance from the invasive tumor front that is *5 mm or more* from the resected margin

Close margin: The distance from the invasive tumor front to the resected margin that is less than 5 mm

Positive margin: Carcinoma-in-situ or invasive carcinoma at the margin of resection

Although the consensus classification of a negative margin is invasive tumor 5 mm or more from the surgical margin, recent evidence suggests that small tumors may not require 5-mm margins, and large tumors may require greater than 5-mm margins to be considered truly negative. Heiduschka and colleagues[15] investigated whether small OSCCs require the same margin clearance as large tumors. They evaluated the association between the ratio of the closest margin to tumor thickness, and correlated their findings with local control and survival. They found that the ratio of margin to tumor thickness was an independent predictor for local recurrence and disease-specific death, and that the minimum safe margin could be calculated by multiplying the tumor thickness by a factor of 0.3 (**Fig. 1**).

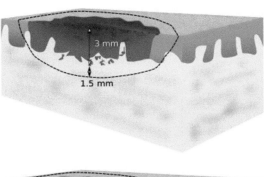

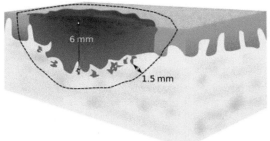

Fig. 1. Two schematized cross-sections of OSCC tumors; tumor thickness was measured as the distance from the level of the mucosa (*dotted line*) to the deepest extent of the tumor. The closest margin in this assumption is between the tumor and the resection (*dashed line*). In the first example, the margin-to–tumor thickness ratio (MTR) is 1.5 mm/3.0 mm = 0.5; in the second example the MTR is 1.5 mm/6.0 mm = 0.25. Hence, a safe margin for a tumor with a thickness of 4 mm requires 1.2 mm, a safe margin for a tumor with 8-mm thickness would be 2.4 mm and a tumor with a thickness of 15 mm would require the traditional margin of 5 mm. (*From* Heiduschka G, Virk SA, Palme CE, et al. Margin to tumor thickness ratio - A predictor of local recurrence and survival in oral squamous cell carcinoma. Oral Oncol 2016;55:49–54; with permission.)

Thus, if the thickness of a given tumor was 5 mm, an adequate resection margin would be merely 1.5 mm. Similarly, if the thickness of a given tumor would be 3 cm, an adequate resection margin would be 10 mm. This concept, although novel, has yet to withstand rigorous scientific evaluation.

SURGICAL MARGIN SHRINKAGE

Obtaining clear margins in OSCC can be challenging due to the difficulty that surgeons often face in navigating the inherent complex and compact anatomy of the oral cavity. When surgeons are able to obtain what appears to be an adequate margin of resection, they are often frustrated to find that the pathologic margin distances are significantly smaller than in situ measurements obtained before resection. Although it is possible that what was thought to have been an adequate margin was actually inadequate, the most common reason for this phenomenon is likely *margin shrinkage*, or the tissue retraction that occurs after resection and pathologic processing of the specimen (**Fig. 2**).

The first study to evaluate margin shrinkage was performed by Johnson and colleagues[16] in 1996. In a study of the oral mucosa of 10 dogs, the investigators found margin shrinkage rates of 30% to 50%. The investigators also noted that most of the shrinkage actually occurred before fixation, suggesting that shrinkage occurs immediately after surgical excision. Subsequent studies of human tissue in patients with OSCC demonstrated margin shrinkage rates ranging from 21% to 75%.[17,18] Tumors located in the buccal mucosa, retro-molar trigone, and mandibular alveolar ridge underwent a significantly greater degree of shrinkage than did tumors of the maxilla and tongue, suggesting that the surgeon consider a wider resection in these areas to aid in achieving a clear surgical margin. There is no clear evidence at this juncture to suggest that tumor stage has an effect on margin shrinkage. Although tissue shrinkage is a confounding factor in obtaining adequate margin diagnoses, margin status discrepancies between frozen and permanent sections are more likely due to increased sampling of the final specimen rather than tissue shrinkage.[18]

INTRAOPERATIVE FROZEN SECTIONS

The surgeon's primary aim is to obtain tumor-free margins of at least 5 mm; however, negative margins are achieved in only 50% to 80% of patients.[19] A technique commonly used by surgeons to assist in obtaining a clear margin is intraoperative frozen section analysis.[20] A recent survey of the International American Head and Neck Society found that more than 97% of head and neck surgeons report the use of intraoperative frozen section analysis in the oral cavity.[21] To obtain a frozen section, fresh tissue specimens embedded in optimal cutting temperature compound are frozen using a cryostat machine, thinly sectioned to an average thickness of approximately 7 μm, and affixed to glass slides. The slides are subsequently fixed, and stained with hematoxylin and eosin, and evaluated by a pathologist.[22] Frozen sections are generally accurate when compared with final surgical margins, with studies reporting accuracy as high as 96% to 98%.[22,23] However, it is important to note that negative intraoperative margins have a substantial false-positive rate ranging from 4% to 14%, and as high as 23% if close margins are considered as well.[22,24,25]

Despite its widespread use, the utility of frozen sections in OSCC is controversial. Frozen sections are costly in terms of time and personnel, with a recent study citing an average cost of more than $3100 per patient.[23] In addition to cost, frozen sectioning often results in oversampling of tissue, which causes increased size of the surgical defect as well as operative time. Finally, there is a dearth

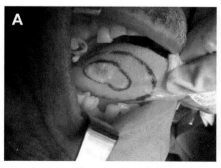
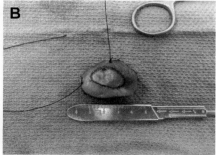

Fig. 2. (*A*) cT1 squamous cell carcinoma of the right lateral tongue, marked circumferentially with a 1-cm margin. (*B*) Same specimen after resection; the greatest degree of margin shrinkage is noted near the floor of the mouth.

of evidence in the literature to support the use of frozen sections when important outcomes, such as final margin status and survival are considered.

It is unclear whether intraoperative frozen section analysis in OSCC is useful in determining final margin status, local recurrence, and disease-specific survival. Gerber and colleagues[26] studied 178 patients with OSCC over a 10-year period who were surgically treated with curative intention, of which 111 patients had frozen sections sent for evaluation. The investigators found that frozen sections did not have any statistically significant impact on final margin status. Pathak and colleagues[27] studied 416 cases of biopsy-proven previously untreated OSCC, of which 55% of patients underwent frozen section analysis during surgical resection. The investigators found that the chance of achieving clear margins was not significantly improved by the use of frozen sections, and the use of frozen sections did not independently predict local recurrence or survival. Although similar findings have been reported by other investigators as well,[13,28] there is recent evidence to suggest that frozen section margins do correlate with local recurrence. A recent retrospective study of 400 patients with OSCC demonstrated that positive margins on frozen sections correlated with a local recurrence rate of 36%, whereas negative frozen margins had a local recurrence rate of 19%.[29]

Because positive margin status on final pathology strongly correlates with local recurrence and poor survival,[30] frozen sections may give the surgeon an additional opportunity to prevent an ultimately positive margin. DiNardo and colleagues[23] reported that 5% of patients in their study of 80 consecutive patients undergoing head and neck malignancy resection were found to have positive margins and benefited from immediate re-resection. In a study of head and neck squamous cell carcinoma resection performed by Du and colleagues,[22] 23% of patients had close or positive margins identified intraoperatively, further resection was performed, and the final margin status was negative. A similar study performed by Ribiero and colleagues[31] found that nearly 90% of patients who had initial positive margins on frozen sections that were re-resected had eventual negative margins on final pathology.

Although frozen sections may afford the surgeon the opportunity to prevent an ultimately positive margin, there is continued debate regarding the effectiveness of this practice. There are those who question if it is realistically feasible for the surgeon to accurately reorient oneself to the "positive" surgical field and resect the remaining tumor. Kerawala and Ong[32] studied this query. In their study, a single surgeon was asked to identify the sites of proposed sampling in 14 consecutive cases of oropharyngeal carcinoma. After approximately 5 minutes, the same surgeon was asked to relocate each site. The study found that the mean error in relocating the sample site was *9 mm* for those placed at mucosal margins and *greater than a centimeter* for samples placed deep to the tumor bed. In 32% of cases, the error was greater than 1 cm.[32] Additional studies by 2 independent groups of head and neck surgeons found that up to 78% of revised margins did not contain *any* residual tumor, suggesting that a large number of revised margins may be routinely taken from a nonrepresentative area.[33,34]

In addition to the difficulty that surgeons have with sample reorientation, the status of improved local recurrence rate and overall survival of patients who undergo revision of positive frozen sections remains questionable. There are a number of studies that suggest that once an initial positive margin is obtained, re-revision to negative may not portend a better overall prognosis for the patient. One retrospective study of 156 patients with head and neck squamous cell carcinoma revealed that local recurrence was strongly associated with positive margins in initial frozen section analysis; 42% of the patients with positive to negative revised tumor margins developed local tumor recurrence compared with 16% local recurrence in the patients with initial tumor-free margins.[35] Guillemaud and colleagues[36] conducted a retrospective chart review of 65 patients and found that both local control and disease-specific survival were significantly reduced in patients who had initial positive frozen sections despite revision to negative. They also found that microscopic tumor cut-through on intraoperative frozen sections independently predicted poorer local control and disease-specific survival, suggesting that positive intraoperative margins simply represent more biologically aggressive disease.

Although there is substantial evidence to suggest that revision of initially positive intraoperative margins may not improve the local recurrence rate and overall survival, there is evidence to suggest that revision of positive margins may improve outcomes in select situations. In a study conducted by Patel and colleagues,[37] 547 patients with OSCC who underwent resection with intraoperative frozen sections were divided into 2 groups. Group 1 had margins that were clear on frozen and permanent sections, whereas group 2 had positive margins on frozen sections that were revised to negative margins on both frozen sections and final pathology. They found that patients *without nodal disease* who had initial positive frozen sections revised to negative margins had disease-specific survival similar to patients with negative frozen sections and final pathology.

FROZEN SECTIONS: DEFECT-DRIVEN VERSUS SPECIMEN-DRIVEN

An essential component of the discussion of intraoperative margin assessment is the tissue-sampling mechanism. A survey conducted in 2005 by Black and colleagues[38] found that most surgeons send fragments of tissue from the surgical bed to be read as frozen sections. Although this "defect-driven" approach is certainly faster and provides the surgeon with precision with regard to specimen site and size, there are several important limitations. Most notably, it is impossible to assess the distance of the surgical margin from the tumor cells because the specimen is submitted with the expectation that the tissue is negative for carcinoma. As such, only involvement of cancer or lack thereof is discernable. In addition, it may be difficult for the pathologist to identify small clusters of tumor cells in these specimens because the known position of tumor bulk is absent from the specimens. These limitations have led surgeons and pathologists alike to conclude that a "specimen-driven approach" to intraoperative frozen section analysis is more accurate, and thus preferred whenever possible. In the "specimen-driven" approach, tissue is sampled from the resected specimen, and the margin distance from the invasive front of the tumor to the resected front is measured.

The advantages of intraoperative sampling via a specimen-driven approach are well documented, and include improved accuracy of final margin status, a reduced rate of local recurrence, and patient survival. A recent prospective randomized controlled trial found that 45% of patients undergoing surgical resection of OSCC had close or positive final margins with patient-driven margins, compared with only 16% of patients with specimen-driven margins, with a sensitivity of 91%.[18] In addition to improved final margin status, Chang and colleagues[34] and Maxwell and colleagues[39] independently observed a significantly reduced rate of local recurrence when specimen-driven margins are used. The difference between the specimen-driven group and the defect-driven group was significant to the point that one investigator declared that defect-driven margins "have no prognostic value."[34] In a prospective pilot study, Yahalom and colleagues[40] found that frozen section sampling from the resected specimen correlated best with final margin status, local recurrence, and overall patient survival. Patients who had negative intraoperative frozen sections sampled from the defect demonstrated a 40% rate of positive margins on final pathology as compared with just 17% in those patients who had specimen-driven margins. In addition, 50% of patients in the defect-driven group developed local recurrence, whereas none of the patients in the specimen-driven group developed local recurrence. Finally, the specimen-driven group had a 100% overall survival rate at the time of the study's publication, as opposed to a 75% survival rate in the defect-driven group.

THE USE OF BIOMARKERS IN EVALUATING THE SURGICAL MARGIN

The principle of "field cancerization" was first presented by Slaughter and colleagues[41] in 1953 when they published the theory that head and neck squamous cell carcinoma arises from swaths of genetically damaged, or as they termed it, "condemned mucosa." The theory was meant to explain the development of multiple primary tumors as well as locally recurrent squamous cell carcinoma in the oral cavity. When considering surgical margins, the notion of field cancerization may be useful in explaining tumor recurrence in the presence of a "complete" surgical excision with negative margins.[42] Although the tissue may appear normal phenotypically, it may have undergone genetic alteration beyond the excised margin that is not visible to the pathologist histologically. A fascinating study by Thomson[43] demonstrated that field cancerization may be a fairly common phenomenon. In his study, 26 consecutive new patients presenting with a unilateral OSCC or a premalignant lesion underwent "mirror image" biopsies from clinically normal-looking mucosa at corresponding anatomic sites. He found that nearly 58% of patients demonstrated histologically abnormal tissue on microscopic examination, including cellular atypia, frank dysplasia, carcinoma-in-situ, or invasive squamous cell carcinoma.[43]

In light of the disturbing trend of local recurrence despite "adequate" histologic surgical excision, researchers have turned to biochemical analysis of the surgical margin to help characterize the true status of the margin, with efforts focused on both molecular genetics and epigenetics. Brennan and colleagues[30] were the first to investigate the presence of an altered p53 gene at histologically normal surgical margins in OSCC. In more than half of the patients who were studied, molecular analysis was positive for a p53 mutation in at least one margin. Thirty-eight percent of those with an altered p53 gene developed local recurrence, as opposed to none of the patients who did not possess the alteration. Subsequently, a study by Nathan and colleagues[44] investigated the presence of eIF4E at histologically negative surgical margins. eIF4E is a well-known proto-oncogene that is activated in nearly all head and neck squamous cell carcinoma. They found that 55% of patients had elevated levels of eIF4E in histologically negative margins and 56% of those patients subsequently developed local recurrence. Only 7% of patients with eIF4E-negative margins developed local recurrence. Subsequent studies have identified additional mutated tumor suppressor genes correlated with local recurrence despite negative margins, including p15, p16, and 9p21.[45,46]

In addition to genetic mutations of both tumor suppressor genes and proto-oncogenes, alterations in gene promoter methylation patterns also have been investigated. In one study, any 2-gene methylation combinations among the genes DCC, EDNRB, and HOXA9 were associated with decreased locoregional recurrence-free survival, recurrence-free survival, and overall survival.[47] Although researchers are aware of a variety of biomarkers that may allow for enhanced characterization of seemingly negative margins, there are very few real-time assays at this juncture that allow for intraoperative detection of biomarkers. Goldenberg and colleagues[48] developed an assay using the quantitative methylation-specific polymerase chain reaction protocol that allows for the detection of methylation-positive margins in less than 5 hours, which could be useful in select major oral squamous cell resection cases that require combined primary tumor resection, cervical lymphadenectomy, and complex reconstruction. As additional real-time biochemical assays are developed for margin analysis, we may be able to obtain true "negative margins" and improve locoregional control and patient survival.

MARGIN STATUS AND ADJUVANT THERAPY

Postoperative adjuvant therapy is often used in treating OSSC to maximize locoregional control in patients with close and positive margins; however, there is no standardized treatment protocol for its use. Although positive margin status correlates negatively with locoregional control, the decision to use adjuvant therapy is usually based on a consideration of multiple factors, including final margin status, degree of nodal disease, tumor thickness, evidence of extranodal and perineural invasion, and lymphovascular spread. It is generally accepted that, if possible, re-resection of the residual carcinoma should be attempted, as the

salvage rate after re-resection is 57% versus 25% if radiotherapy is performed alone.[6,49]

The most commonly used adjuvant therapy is postoperative radiotherapy (PORT). Although the use of PORT has been demonstrated to improve disease-free survival and local control in patients with close and positive margins, its use must be balanced against its morbidity. In general, PORT is not considered to be of benefit in treating early-stage disease (stage I-II) that has been resected with negative margins. PORT is generally recommended for patients with advanced disease (stage III-IV), or disease of any stage with positive margins.

There has been a surge in interest in the use of adjuvant chemotherapy in the treatment of OSCC. In 1997, the first trial investigating the use of both chemotherapy and radiotherapy in treating margin-positive OSCC was conducted by the Radiation Therapy Oncology Group (RTOG).[50] The RTOG 88 to 24 trial demonstrated a 55% risk reduction when cisplatin and radiotherapy were combined, and was the first study to demonstrate improved locoregional disease control with adjuvant chemo-radiotherapy versus radiotherapy alone. The results of this study gave rise to 2 large prospective randomized controlled trials that confirmed that adjuvant chemo-radiation is more efficacious in treating margin-positive OSCC than adjuvant radiotherapy alone. The first study, known as RTOG 9501, demonstrated that when residual tumor is located at the surgical margin, the estimated 2-year locoregional control rate was 82% in the combined chemo-radiotherapy group, as opposed to 72% in the radiotherapy group.[51] The study also found that the combination of adjuvant chemotherapy and radiotherapy in margin-positive OSCC resulted in a significant increase in disease-free survival; however, overall survival was not significantly improved. The second trial was conducted by the European Organization for Research and Treatment of Cancer (EORTC) and published the same year as the RTOG 9501 trial. The EORTC trial demonstrated that the rate of both disease-free survival *and* overall survival were significantly higher in the chemo-radiotherapy group than in the radiotherapy cohort alone.[52] An important distinction between this study and the RTOG 9501 study is that in the EORTC trial a positive margin was classified as carcinoma *less than 5 mm* from the surgical margin, which suggests that patients with close, but not necessarily positive margins also were included. A retrospective subgroup analysis of the 2 trials found that adjuvant chemo-radiotherapy improved outcomes in margin-positive squamous cell carcinoma,[53] and the current recommendation of the NCCN is that patients with extracapsular nodal spread and/or positive surgical margins receive adjuvant chemo-radiotherapy.[6]

Although the benefit of adjuvant chemo-radiotherapy for margin-positive OSCC is clear, the role of adjuvant therapy in the case of a "close" (>1 mm, <5 mm) margin remains unclear, and as is the case with positive margins, there is a lack of a postoperative standardized treatment protocol when managing close margins. The implication of the EORTC trial is that despite the added toxicity, a "close margin" should be treated with adjuvant chemo-radiotherapy to improve locoregional control and survival. However, the results of a recent retrospective study performed by Ch'ng and colleagues[54] appear to demonstrate that surgery alone is sufficient in the treatment of close margins, and that the local control rate for all patients who underwent surgery alone was 91%, and the disease-specific survival rate was 84% at 5 years. Although this study appears to suggest that surgery alone is sufficient in the treatment of close margins, some have raised doubts regarding the reliability of the data. It has been pointed out that the investigators failed to exclude patients who underwent margin revision after positive margins were initially obtained on frozen sections.[55] As discussed earlier, regardless of final margin status, a positive intraoperative margin is suggestive of more aggressive disease and thus the inclusion of such patients in the study may limit the generalizability of the study's results. Due to the lack of conclusive evidence regarding the role of adjuvant therapy in managing close surgical margins, it is recommended that one consider additional adverse parameters, such as extranodal extension, tumor thickness, and angio-lymphatic invasion.

A final consideration in the treatment of both close and positive margins in OSCC is the use of brachytherapy. Brachytherapy, or interstitial radiotherapy, allows for the insertion of a radioactive source either adjacent to or directly into the tumor mass. Local control rates of up to 93% have been demonstrated in patients with close or positive margins treated by ^{192}Ir brachytherapy after adjuvant radiotherapy.[56] Chao and colleagues[57] studied patients who were treated with brachytherapy for T1 or T2 tongue and floor-of-mouth squamous cell carcinoma, and found that patients with positive margins treated with brachytherapy had a comparable rate of local control to patients with negative margins treated solely with radiotherapy. Lapeyre and colleagues[58] advocate that brachytherapy replace radiotherapy in T1/T2 lesions with close and positive margins, as they

found equivalent survival and local control rates in both groups, with decreased rates of xerostomia and other adverse effects of adjuvant radiotherapy.

REFERENCES

1. Siegel RL, Miller KD, Jemal A. Cancer statistics, 2016. CA Cancer J Clin 2016;66(1):7–30.
2. Ermer MA, Kirsch K, Bittermann G, et al. Recurrence rate and shift in histopathological differentiation of oral squamous cell carcinoma–a long-term retrospective study over a period of 13.5 years. J Craniomaxillofac Surg 2015;43(7):1309–13.
3. Liao CT, Chang JT, Wang HM, et al. Analysis of risk factors of predictive local tumor control in oral cavity cancer. Ann Surg Oncol 2008;15(3):915–22.
4. Chen TY, Emrich LJ, Driscoll DL. The clinical significance of pathological findings in surgically resected margins of the primary tumor in head and neck carcinoma. Int J Radiat Oncol Biol Phys 1987;13(6):833–7.
5. Lin YT, Chien CY, Lu CT, et al. Triple-positive pathologic findings in oral cavity cancer are related to a dismal prognosis. Laryngoscope 2015;125(9):E300–5.
6. NCCN-Principles of surgery-Margins SURG-A v1.2015, National Comprehensive Cancer Network Inc. Head and Neck Cancers.
7. Kurita H, Nakanishi Y, Nishizawa R, et al. Impact of different surgical margin conditions on local recurrence of oral squamous cell carcinoma. Oral Oncol 2010;46(11):814–7.
8. Sutton DN, Brown JS, Rogers SN, et al. The prognostic implications of the surgical margin in oral squamous cell carcinoma. Int J Oral Maxillofac Surg 2003;32(1):30–4.
9. Loree TR, Strong EW. Significance of positive margins in oral cavity squamous carcinoma. Am J Surg 1990;160(4):410–4.
10. Yamada S, Kurita H, Shimane T, et al. Estimation of the width of free margin with a significant impact on local recurrence in surgical resection of oral squamous cell carcinoma. Int J Oral Maxillofac Surg 2016;45(2):147–52.
11. Anderson CR, Sisson K, Moncrieff M. A meta-analysis of margin size and local recurrence in oral squamous cell carcinoma. Oral Oncol 2015;51(5):464–9.
12. Looser KG, Shah JP, Strong EW. The significance of positive margins in surgically resected epidermoid carcinomas. Head Neck Surg 1978;1(2):107–11.
13. Binahmed A, Nason RW, Abdoh AA. The clinical significance of the positive surgical margin in oral cancer. Oral Oncol 2007;43(8):780–4.
14. Dik EA, Willems SM, Ipenburg NA, et al. Resection of early oral squamous cell carcinoma with positive or close margins: relevance of adjuvant

treatment in relation to local recurrence: margins of 3 mm as safe as 5 mm. Oral Oncol 2014;50(6): 611–5.

15. Heiduschka G, Virk SA, Palme CE, et al. Margin to tumor thickness ratio–a predictor of local recurrence and survival in oral squamous cell carcinoma. Oral Oncol 2016;55:49–54.

16. Johnson RE, Sigman JD, Funk GF, et al. Quantification of surgical margin shrinkage in the oral cavity. Head Neck 1997;19(4):281–6.

17. Mistry RC, Qureshi SS, Kumaran C. Post-resection mucosal margin shrinkage in oral cancer: quantification and significance. J Surg Oncol 2005; 91(2):131–3.

18. Cheng A, Cox D, Schmidt BL. Oral squamous cell carcinoma margin discrepancy after resection and pathologic processing. J Oral Maxillofac Surg 2008;66(3):523–9.

19. Amit M, Na'ara S, Leider-Trejo L, et al. Improving the rate of negative margins after surgery for oral cavity squamous cell carcinoma: a prospective randomized controlled study. Head Neck 2015;38(Suppl 1):E1803–9.

20. Wenig BM. Intraoperative consultation (IOC) in mucosal lesions of the upper aerodigestive tract. Head Neck Pathol 2008;2(2):131–44.

21. Meier JD, Oliver DA, Varvares MA. Surgical margin determination in head and neck oncology: current clinical practice. The results of an International American Head and Neck Society Member Survey. Head & neck 2005;27(11):952–8.

22. Du E, Ow TJ, Lo YT, et al. Refining the utility and role of frozen section in head and neck squamous cell carcinoma resection. Laryngoscope 2016;126(8): 1768–75.

23. DiNardo LJ, Lin J, Karageorge LS, et al. Accuracy, utility, and cost of frozen section margins in head and neck cancer surgery. Laryngoscope 2000; 110(10):1773–6.

24. Spiro RH, Guillamondegui O Jr, Paulino AF, et al. Pattern of invasion and margin assessment in patients with oral tongue cancer. Head & neck 1999; 21(5):408–13.

25. Ord RA, Aisner S. Accuracy of frozen sections in assessing margins in oral cancer resection. J Oral Maxillofac Surg 1997;55(7):663–9.

26. Gerber S, Gengler C, Grätz KW, et al. The impact of frozen sections on final surgical margins in squamous cell carcinoma of the oral cavity and lips: a retrospective analysis over an 11 years period. Head Neck Oncol 2011;3(1):1.

27. Pathak KA, Nason RW, Penner C, et al. Impact of use of frozen section assessment of operative margins on survival in oral cancer. Oral Surg Oral Med Oral Pathol Oral Radiol Endod 2009;107(2):235–9.

28. Nason RW, Binahmed A, Pathak KA, et al. What is the adequate margin of surgical resection in oral cancer? Oral Surg Oral Med Oral Pathol Oral Radiol Endodontology 2009;107(5):625–9.

29. Buchakjian MR, Tasche KK, Robinson RA, et al. Association of main specimen and tumor bed margin status with local recurrence and survival in oral cancer surgery. JAMA Otolaryngol Head Neck Surg 2016;142(12):1191–8.

30. Brennan JA, Mao L, Hruban RH, et al. Molecular assessment of histopathological staging in squamous-cell carcinoma of the head and neck. N Engl J Med 1995;332(7):429–35.

31. Ribeiro NFF, Godden DR, Wilson GE, et al. Do frozen sections help achieve adequate surgical margins in the resection of oral carcinoma? Int J Oral Maxillofac Surg 2003;32(2):152–8.

32. Kerawala CJ, Ong TK. Relocating the site of frozen sections—is there room for improvement? Head & neck 2001;23(3):230–2.

33. Scholl P, Byers RM, Batsakis JG, et al. Microscopic cut-through of cancer in the surgical treatment of squamous carcinoma of the tongue: prognostic and therapeutic implications. Am J Surg 1986; 152(4):354–60.

34. Chang AMV, Kim SW, Duvvuri U, et al. Early squamous cell carcinoma of the oral tongue: comparing margins obtained from the glossectomy specimen to margins from the tumor bed. Oral Oncol 2013; 49(11):1077–82.

35. Ettl T, El-Gindi A, Hautmann M, et al. Positive frozen section margins predict local recurrence in R0-resected squamous cell carcinoma of the head and neck. Oral Oncol 2016;55:17–23.

36. Guillemaud JP, Patel RS, Goldstein DP, et al. Prognostic impact of intraoperative microscopic cut-through on frozen section in oral cavity squamous cell carcinoma. J Otolaryngol Head Neck Surg 2010;39(4):370–7.

37. Patel RS, Goldstein DP, Guillemaud J, et al. Impact of positive frozen section microscopic tumor cut-through revised to negative on oral carcinoma control and survival rates. Head Neck 2010;32(11): 1444–51.

38. Black C, Marotti J, Zarovnaya E, et al. Critical evaluation of frozen section margins in head and neck cancer resections. Cancer 2006;107(12): 2792–800.

39. Maxwell JH, Thompson LD, Brandwein-Gensler MS, et al. Early oral tongue squamous cell carcinoma: sampling of margins from tumor bed and worse local control. JAMA Otolaryngol Head Neck Surg 2015;141(12):1–8.

40. Yahalom R, Dobriyan A, Vered M, et al. A prospective study of surgical margin status in oral squamous cell carcinoma: a preliminary report. J Surg Oncol 2008; 98:572–8.

41. Slaughter DP, Southwick HW, Smejkal W. "Field cancerization" in oral stratified squamous epithelium.

Clinical implications of multicentric origin. Cancer 1953;6(5):963–8.

42. Westra WH, Sidransky D. Phenotypic and genotypic disparity in premalignant lesions: of calm water and crocodiles. J Natl Cancer Inst 1998;90(20):1500–1.

43. Thomson PJ. Field change and oral cancer: new evidence for widespread carcinogenesis? Int J Oral Maxillofac Surg 2002;31(3):262–6.

44. Nathan CO, Franklin S, Abreo FW, et al. Analysis of surgical margins with the molecular marker eIF4E: a prognostic factor in patients with head and neck cancer. J Clin Oncol 1999;17(9):2909–14.

45. Hayashi M, Wu G, Roh JL, et al. Correlation of gene methylation in surgical margin imprints with locoregional recurrence in head and neck squamous cell carcinoma. Cancer 2015;121:1957–65.

46. Wang X, Chen S, Chen X, et al. Tumor-related markers in histologically normal margins correlate with locally recurrent oral squamous cell carcinoma: a retrospective study. J Oral Pathol Med 2016;45(2):83–8.

47. Graveland AP, Golusinski PJ, Buijze M, et al. Loss of heterozygosity at 9p and p53 immunopositivity in surgical margins predict local relapse in head and neck squamous cell carcinoma. Int J Cancer 2011; 128(8):1852–9.

48. Goldenberg D, Harden S, Masayesva BG, et al. Intraoperative molecular margin analysis in head and neck cancer. Arch Otolaryngol Head Neck Surg 2004;130(1):39–44.

49. Brown JS, Shaw RJ, Bekiroglu F, et al. Systematic review of the current evidence in the use of postoperative radiotherapy for oral squamous cell carcinoma. Br J Oral Maxillofac Surg 2012;50(6):481–9.

50. Al-Sarraf M, Pajak TF, Byhardt RW, et al. Postoperative radiotherapy with concurrent cisplatin appears to improve locoregional control of advanced, resectable head and neck cancers: RTOG 88-24. Int J Radiat Oncol Biol Phys 1997;37(4):777.

51. Cooper JS, Pajak TF, Forastiere AA, et al. Postoperative concurrent radiotherapy and chemotherapy for high-risk squamous-cell carcinoma of the head and neck. N Engl J Med 2004;350: 1937–44.

52. Bernier J, Domenge C, Ozsahin M, et al. Postoperative irradiation with or without concomitant chemotherapy for locally advanced head and neck cancer. N Engl J Med 2004;350: 1945–52.

53. Bernier J, Cooper JS, Pajak TF, et al. Defining risk levels in locally advanced head and neck cancers: a comparative analysis of concurrent postoperative radiation plus chemotherapy trials of the EORTC (#22931) and RTOG (# 9501). Head Neck 2005;27: 843–50.

54. Ch'ng S, Corbett-Burns S, Stanton N, et al. Close margin alone does not warrant postoperative adjuvant radiotherapy in oral squamous cell carcinoma. Cancer 2013;119:2427–37.

55. Duvvuri U, Seethala RR, Chiosea S. Margin assessment in oral squamous cell carcinoma. Cancer 2014;120:452–3.

56. Beitler JJ, Smith RV, Silver CE, et al. Close or positive margins after surgical resection for the head and neck cancer patient: the addition of brachytherapy improves local control. Int J Radiat Oncol Biol Phys 1998;40:313–7.

57. Chao KS, Emami B, Akhileswaran R, et al. The impact of surgical margin status and use of an interstitial implant on T1, T2 oral tongue cancers after surgery. Int J Radiat Oncol Biol Phys 1996;36: 1039–43.

58. Lapeyre M, Bollet MA, Racadot S, et al. Postoperative brachytherapy alone and combined postoperative radiotherapy and brachytherapy boost for squamous cell carcinoma of the oral cavity, with positive or close margins. Head Neck 2004;26: 216–23.

Margin Analysis
Squamous Cell Carcinoma of the Oropharynx

Felix W. Sim, MBBS, BDS, MFDS(Eng), FRACDS(OMS)[a],
Hong D. Xiao, MD, PhD[b], R. Bryan Bell, MD, DDS[a],*

KEYWORDS

- Surgical margins • Oropharyngeal cancer • Squamous cell carcinoma • Prognosis • Local control
- Head and neck • HPV

KEY POINTS

- Oropharyngeal carcinoma should now be considered as a distinct subsite of head and neck carcinoma because of the distinct biological differences and response to treatment.
- There seems to be a consistently favorable outcome not only in survival but also locoregional control of human papilloma virus–positive oropharyngeal squamous cell carcinoma.
- Special optical imaging devices (eg, narrow band imaging) have been used for better delineation of surgical margins resulting in lower rates of positive margins.
- Molecular assessment of margins is still evolving and not yet clinically practical for everyday use of margin assessment; but in the era of immunotherapy, there is ongoing research to determine the markers that can be used to predict responders to nonresponders of immunotherapy.

INTRODUCTION

Surgical margins have been an ongoing topic of discussion in head and neck surgery. It is well accepted that close or positive margins are related to increased risk of locoregional recurrence. In their review of surgical margins in head and neck cancer, Alicandri-Ciufelli and colleagues[1] confirmed that inadequate surgical resection margins contribute to increased local recurrence and decreased survival rates.

The oropharynx includes the segment of the pharynx from the level of the hard palate down to the hyoid bone. Anatomically, it is composed of the base of the tongue, palatine tonsil, soft palate, and lateral and posterior pharyngeal wall. Worldwide, there are more than 400,000 new cases of oropharyngeal carcinoma per year with nearly 46,000 new cases in the United States alone.[2] Most of these carcinomas are squamous cell carcinomas (SCCs). Historically and up to this day, because of the common shared risk factors of smoking and heavy alcohol consumption, literature involving oropharyngeal SCC (OPSCC) is often combined with oral SCC. However, since the introduction of a link between human papilloma virus (HPV) and OPSCC more than 15 years ago,[3,4] HPV is now confirmed to be a major risk factor of OPSCC with its distinct epidemiology and favorable treatment outcome; there is a need to consider OPSCC separate from the other subsites of head and neck SCC. Two recent meta-analyses by Petrelli and colleagues[5] and O'Rorke and colleagues[6] both confirm a survival advantage

The authors have nothing to disclose.
[a] Head and Neck Institute, Providence Cancer Center, Providence Portland Medical Center, 4805 Northeast Glisan Street, Suite 6N50, Portland, OR 97213, USA; [b] Head and Neck Pathologist, Department of Pathology, Providence Portland Medical Center, 4805 Northeast Glisan Street, Suite 6N50, Portland, OR 97213, USA
* Corresponding author.
E-mail address: richard.bell@providence.org

oralmaxsurgery.theclinics.com

for patients with HPV-positive head and neck carcinoma as compared with those with HPV-negative disease (hazard ratio [HR] 0.46; 95% confidence interval [CI], 0.37–0.57 and HR = 0.33; 95% CI, 0.27–0.40, respectively). Excess tobacco use is shown to be have a negative influence, as patients with HPV-positive head and neck cancer and significant tobacco use histories have outcomes intermediate to those in HPV-positive nonsmokers or traditional HPV-negative (ie, tobacco and/or alcohol associated) head and neck cancers.[7,8] The incidence of larynx, oral cavity, and hypopharynx SCC is declining, whereas the incidence of OPSCCs, particularly in the tonsillar and base of tongue region, have demonstrated a recent increase in incidence in the United States, Canada, Australia, Denmark, Japan, Slovakia, and the United Kingdom.[9] Patients with HP-positive OPSCC are usually nonsmokers, male, and younger with a median age of 58 years compared with the median age of 63 years for classic smoker- and drinker-related OPSCC.[9,10]

Before the advent of sophisticated radiation techniques and transoral laser and robotic surgery, OPSCC was managed surgically via invasive lip split mandibulotomy to gain access to the base of the tongue and palatine tonsil with subsequent reconstruction of the defect with a vascularized free flap.[11,12] Most of these patients still required adjuvant radiation therapy. In the effort to improve function and minimize morbidity of surgery, definitive radiotherapy was shown to be an effective method of treating stage I and II OPSCC with 5-year local control, regional control, locoregional control, and disease-free survival (DFS) rates of 85%, 93%, 81%, and 77%, respectively.[13] An Eastern Cooperative Oncology Group (E2399) clinical trial examining the addition of induction and concurrent paclitaxel chemotherapy to the radiation regime showed reduction of the 2-year local failure rate of stage III and IV OPSCC to 16% with a 2-year overall survival rate of 83%.[14] In 2002, a meta-analysis of patients with OPSCC found equivalent survival outcomes for patients treated with surgery and adjuvant radiotherapy versus definitive radiotherapy with salvage neck dissection. It also found that there was a significant difference in severe complications between the two cohorts favoring definitive radiotherapy.[15] Despite this effectiveness, chemoradiation is still associated with significant long-term toxicity and functional impairment.[16,17] Up until 2009, in most countries in the world, primary radiation with or without chemotherapy is still the main treatment option for OPSCC.

SURGICAL TREATMENT OF OROPHARYNGEAL SQUAMOUS CELL CARCINOMA

With the improved outcomes to radiotherapy of HPV-related OPSCC as elucidated earlier, and the never-ending quest of providing the most effective treatment with the least morbidity, there has been a recent paradigm shift of the management of early OPSCC toward minimally invasive transoral surgery. This review focuses on the analysis of margins obtained by these minimally invasive surgical treatments.

Transoral Laser Microsurgery

Transoral laser microsurgery (TLM) is not a novel concept and was introduced by Steiner and colleagues[18,19] for the management of laryngeal and piriform sinus carcinomas over the last couple of decades. The same investigators described the use of TLM for OPSCC in 2003.[20] In this same period, TLM has gained popularity in centers in the United Kingdom and the United States as an alternative surgical option because of the reduced cost compared with transoral robotic surgery (TORS) and reported superior functional outcomes.[21,22]

TLM is performed under suspended direct laryngoscopy and an operating microscope to expose and visualize the tumor. Resection is then carried out with a carbon dioxide (CO_2) laser. One key principle of TLM as described by Steiner and colleagues[20] that distinguishes it from other surgical treatment is that the tumor is transected at its most proximal portion with the CO_2 laser to estimate the depth of invasion. The primary tumor is then completely resected in multiple blocs to achieve tumor-free surgical margins. Large tumors are transected and cored out to reduce their size, allowing resection of the remaining shell of tumor using a series of transtumoral cuts.

Transoral Robotic Surgery

Weinstein and colleagues[23] reported the first case series using the da Vinci Surgical System (Intuitive Surgical, Inc, Sunnyvale, California) for radical tonsillectomy. After 4 phases of clinical trials confirming the safety, efficacy, and cost-effectiveness, in 2009, the US Food and Drug Administration approved the da Vinci Surgical System for TORS.

For a TORS case, patients are intubated orally with a reinforced endotracheal tube, which is sutured to the contralateral buccal mucosa. Patients are rotated 180° away from the anesthesiologist. The patients' eyes are protected using an adhesive plastic eye shield, and the maxillary teeth are often protected with a dental guard.

Specialized oral retractors are placed (eg, Crowe-Davis retractor) and rigidly secured to the operating table for optimal surgical exposure and visualization. Proper placement and fixation of the retractor are critical for success in TORS. The robot is docked at a 30° to 45° angle to the operating table. The camera arm is then positioned centrally; arms 1 and 2 are positioned on either side of the camera arm, allowing optimal range of movement with minimal collisions. A variety of different instruments can be used to grasp, cut, and dissect the tumor from the surrounding oropharyngeal tissue (eg, monopolar electrocautery, Maryland dissector forceps, or CO_2). An assistant is positioned at the patients' head to provide retraction and suction during the procedure.

Specifically, for OPSCC, TORS have been limited to T1 and T2 primaries, as the ability to obtain a negative margin is one of the key indications for TORS in managing OPSCC[24] (**Fig. 1**). Unlike TLM whereby the tumor is resected piecemeal, a TORS resection principle is removed stepwise with constant anatomically defined cuts. As per the original description by Weinstein and colleagues[23] and O'Malley and colleagues,[25] the resected specimen is orientated and brought to the pathologist for inspection. If the surgeon and pathologist agree that margins were grossly negative for tumor, then no frozen sections are obtained and the specimen is processed for permanent margins. However, if the margins seem questionable, then sections are frozen to assess these margins. Positive margins identified on frozen sections will allow the surgeon to remove additional soft tissue margin in the area of question.

BIOLOGICAL DIFFERENCE OF HUMAN PAPILLOMA VIRUS–POSITIVE AND NEGATIVE OROPHARYNGEAL SQUAMOUS CELL CARCINOMA

Discussion about surgical margins must include the biological difference of HPV-positive versus HPV-negative OPSCC to better understand the difference in treatment response and reduced locoregional recurrence rate despite surgical clearance often achieving margins less than what is deemed to be clear in other subsites of the head and neck (5 mm or greater). HPV-negative OPSCCs are more similar to conventional tobacco- and alcohol-related SCC with high p53 mutation rate and are more likely to have an increased epidermal growth factor receptor expression by immunohistochemistry.[26]

In HPV-positive OPSCC, the most common viral genotypes found are HPV 16, 18, and 33. HPV

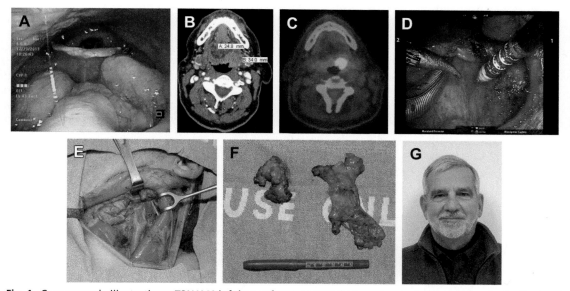

Fig. 1. Case example illustrating a T2N1M0 left base of tongue SCC that was treated with TORS and selective level 2 to 4 neck dissection. (*A*) Tumor viewed from direct nasopharyngoscopy showing ulcerated mass occupying left base of tongue and glosso-tonsillar sulcus with no involvement of vallecula. (*B, C*) Staging computed tomography and PET showing extent of involvement and size of tumor. (*D*) Intraoperative photograph of TORS resection of base of tongue showing superior extent of resection to include lateral pharyngeal wall. (*E*) Following removal of level 2 to 4 nodal tissue with preservation of level 1b. (*F*) Specimen from left tongue base and left neck. (*G*) Patient 3 months following completion of adjuvant radiotherapy for intermediate-risk features.

DNA is 6800 to 8000 base pairs long, which when translated, codes for 8 genes. The genes are broken down into early and late phase, indicating which stage of basal cell infection they are introduced. E1, E2, E4, E5, E6, and E7 make up the early phase genes; L1 and L2 are the late-phase genes. Once the viral DNA is integrated within the keratinocytes, the overexpression of 2 integral genes in the HPV genome are responsible for oncogenesis. The E6 protein inhibits the role of p53, and E7 inhibits the role of the retinoblastoma protein (Rb). Both p53 and Rb are involved in the regulation of cells with damaged/mutated DNA whereby when activated ultimately leads to apoptosis. When E6 protein of HPV binds to the host p53 protein, it causes a structural change and the variant of p53 is no longer able to bind to damaged DNA, thereby inhibiting apoptosis. The Rb gene codes for a protein that restricts cell replication. When the E7 protein binds to and degrades Rb protein, it is no longer functional and cell proliferation is left unchecked[27] (**Fig. 2**).

Toll like receptors (TLRs) have been implicated in cancer development, and there is some suggestion that HPV induces change in the TLR expression pattern during carcinogenesis of the cervix.[28] Jouhi and colleagues[29] analyzed the differences in the expression patterns of TLRs of HPV-positive and HPV-negative OPSCC and found that there is high TLR 5 expressions in the p16-negative and low TLR 5 expressions in the

p16–positive OPSCC cell line. Activation of TLR 5 has been shown to protect tissue adjacent to tumor from radiation toxicity via secretion of radio-protective cytokines, without reducing the radiosensitivity of the tumor.[30] The investigators hypothesized that high expression of TLR 5 in p16-negative OPSCC may have a protective role on tumor tissue from radiation treatment and, therefore, contribute to the poorer treatment response to radiotherapy. This hypothesis is further supported by similar findings of high TLR 5 expression in oral SCC, which is associated with a worse prognosis and recurrences that is proportional with elevation of TLR 5 expression.[31]

Swick and colleagues[32] reviewed the immunologic difference of HPV-positive tumors, showing that HPV-positive tumors are associated with a more immunologically rich microenvironment that influences the tumor's response to treatment. There are increased numbers of tumor infiltrating lymphocytes (TILs) in HPV-positive tumors,[33] with greater expression of programmed death-1 (PD-1).[34] Patients who have a favorable outcome are shown to have a high CD8 TIL count and low CD4/CD8 ratio confirming the importance of cytotoxic T cells in killing HPV-infected malignant cells. Interestingly, the protein that activates CD8 cells, human leukocyte antigen-1, is paradoxically downregulated in HPV-positive OPSCC leading to a decrease in survival when found in high intensity.[35] There is a shift of the T-cell population

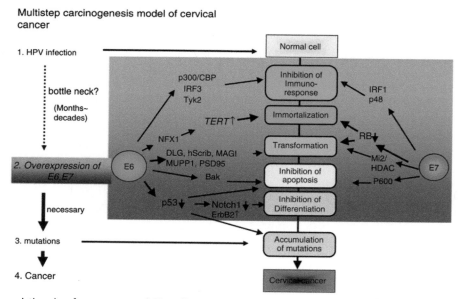

Fig. 2. Synergistic role of overexpressed E6 and E7 gene leading to inactivation of p53 and Rb gene that leads to the cancer. (*From* Narisawa-Saito M, Kiyono T. Basic mechanisms of high-risk human papillomavirus-induced carcinogenesis: roles of E6 and E7 proteins. Cancer Sci 2007;98(10):1506; with permission)

from naïve to memory or effector T cells with greater frequency compared with patients with HPV-negative tumors.[36]

With all the research comparing and contrasting HPV-positive and HPV-negative OPSCC, the mechanisms underlying the clinical differences between the two entities may involve the combined effects of tumor cell intrinsic features and interactions between tumor cells and stromal cells of the activated tumor microenvironment, especially cells of the adaptive and innate immunity.

OUTCOMES OF SURGICAL TREATMENT REGARDING MARGINS

Table 1 summarizes the pertinent articles focusing on OPSCC and does not include those that combine oral and oropharyngeal carcinoma in the study group

The long-held practice of oncologic surgery based on the Halsted principle is strict en bloc resection of primary tumor and a margin of normal-appearing tissue to include all microscopic tumor extension. Although there is agreement that failure to achieve negative margins during resection of the primary tumor increases the likelihood of local recurrence and overall survival,[43,44] there is no universal definition of what constitutes an inadequate resection margin. The guidelines from the American Society of Clinical Oncology (ASCO), National Comprehensive Cancer Network (NCCN), and European Oncology Institute (IEO) define a close margin as 5 mm or less without any subsite distinction. A published survey of members of the American Head and Neck Society, regarding the definition of margins, revealed that the most common cutoff for a clear margin was greater than 5 mm on microscopic examination.[45] Alicandri-Ciufell and colleagues,[1] in their comprehensive review on surgical margins in head and neck, reported that most studies use a margin distance of 5 mm or greater to define margin clearance, with the exception of glottic cancer in which there is a long-standing consensus that resection margins may be as limited as 1 to 2 mm and still be considered adequate. For TORS resection of oropharyngeal tumors, Weinstein and colleagues[40] defined a margin of 2 mm or less to be considered close and anything greater than 2 mm considered a free margin, which has been adopted at the authors' institution (**Fig. 3**).

The incidence of positive tumor margins in OPSCC resected with TORS was 3.8%.[40] These rates compare favorably with other transoral approaches.[39,46] No oncological outcomes were reported in this preliminary study.

A follow-up retrospective study by Weinstein and colleagues[47] analyzed local control from the same population group of 30 patients who had previously untreated OPSCC managed only with TORS. In 30 primary TORS procedures for OPSCC, final pathologic evaluation revealed one case with a positive margin (3%), defined as tumor presence at the inked margin. This patient had focal positivity of carcinoma in situ, and re-excision was performed. The one local recurrence that occurred 3 months following TORS was in a patient with a pT2N0 tumor.[47] This patient had negative margins following TORS, with pathologic analysis showing a poorly differentiated SCC. It is important to note that these retrospective studies did not analyze p16 or HPV status of the specimens.

Cohen and colleagues analyzed 66 patients who underwent TORS as primary therapy for OPSCC with a minimum follow-up of 2 years. In this study, most OPSCCs were p16 positive (89.2%). In 36 patients (54.5%) surgical margins were clear on the initial resection. Of the 30 patients who had positive margins on initial frozen section, 12 patients (18.2%) required a second margin excision at the time of the initial operation and 18 patients (27.3%) required 3 or more margin excisions at the time of the initial operation. One patient with clear margins on frozen section pathologic examination at the initial operation was later found to have carcinoma in situ at one tumor margin on final analysis. The 3-year estimated local control was 97.0%, regional control was 94.0%, and distant control was 98.4%. Disease-specific survival was 95.1%, whereas recurrence-free survival was 92.4%. It is worth noting that with only 54.5% patients having clear margins on initial resection and the remainder requiring additional reresection to achieve clear margins, the local recurrence rate remained very low. The investigators attributed this to the good intraoperative orientation and communication with an experience pathologist. However, with a high percentage of tumors being p16 positive, the favorable outcomes could also be attributed to the different biology and tumor microenvironment (TME) as described previously.

In one of the largest multi-institutional studies of the outcomes of TORS by de Almeida and colleagues,[42] 88.8% of its population had OPSCC. There were 2 interesting findings on locoregional recurrence and survival data based on HPV status. This study found that HPV status had no impact in locoregional control, overall survival, and disease-specific survival. Locoregional control was significantly affected by the margin status. At the 2-year follow-up, the locoregional control rate for patients with positive margins during TORS was

Table 1
Up-to-date outcome studies on oropharyngeal squamous cell carcinoma, margins, local control, and survival

Author, Year	Sample Size	HPV Status	(%)	Method of Resection	Definition of Close Margins	Positive Margins on Final Pathology	Local Control (%)	Survival Outcome (%)	Study Period
Haughey et al,[21] 2011	204	Positive	74.0	TLM	N/A	7.0% (15 of 204)	96.5	89.0 (OS)	2 y
Cohen et al,[37] 2011	50	Positive	74.0	TORS	≤2 mm	2.0% (1 of 50)	100.0	80.6 (OS)	2 y
Karatzanis et al,[38] 2011	223	N/A	—	TLM, transoral electrocautery	N/A	8.0% (15 of 223)	93.0	88.0 (OS)	5 y
Moore et al,[39] 2009	66	Positive	72.1	TORS	N/A	1.5% (1 of 66)	97.0	92.4 (DFS)	3 y
Weinstein et al,[40] 2012	30	N/A	—	TORS	≤2 mm	1.0% (1 of 30)	97.0	100.0 (OS)	2 y
Ford et al,[41] 2014	65	Positive	81.0	TORS	≤5 mm	10.0% (15 of 65)	N/A	91.0 (OS)	2 y
	65	Positive	79.0	Open	—	12.0% (18 of 65)	N/A	75.0 (OS)	2 y
de Almeida et al,[42] 2015	410	Negative	17.1	TORS	≤5 mm	9.0% (39 of 410)	91.8	91.0 (OS)	1.5 y
	—	Positive	38.8	—	—	—	—	—	—
	—	Unknown	44.1	—	—	—	—	—	—

Abbreviations: N/A, not applicable/recorded; OS, overall survival.

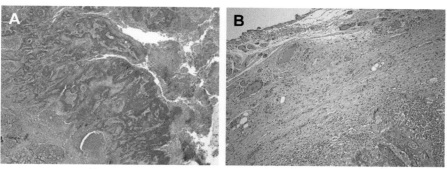

Fig. 3. (*A, B*) Photomicrograph of resection margin of OPSCC showing less than 5 mm clearance (hematoxylin-eosin, original magnification ×100).

78.6% compared with 92.9% when surgical margins were negative. The investigators acknowledged that with no HPV status information on 181 of 410 patients (44.1%), limited conclusions can be drawn on oncologic outcomes based on HPV status.

Iyer and colleagues[48] conducted a detailed retrospective analysis of surgically treated HPV-positive and negative oropharyngeal cancer of 201 patients correlating clinicopathologic factors and 5-year survival outcomes. Consistent with current trends, they found that surgically treated patients with p16-positive oropharyngeal carcinoma have superior survival compared with p16-negative patients. Of interest, supporting the hypothesis that the TME and host immune response may play a key role is their finding that margin status significantly affected disease-specific survival in p16-negative patients while having minimal effect on prognosis in p16-positive patients (**Fig. 4**).

Most of the recent studies that analyzed HPV or p16 status on oncological outcomes of OPSCC in relation to margins do show that there seems to be a consistently favorable outcome not only in survival but also locoregional control of HPV-positive OPSCC.[21,37,49,50] It is not known what

accounts for the more favorable margin control and narrower margin threshold in HPV-related disease as compared with HPV-negative cancers. However, it is speculated that perhaps the immune response to viral epitopes contributes to antitumor immunity and better margin control. Recent use of multi-spectrum imaging and immunofluorescence for qualitative and quantitative assessment of the TME at the invasive margin/resection margins and stroma may provide some insight into this question moving forward (**Fig. 5**). Regardless, the fact that narrow margin resection seems to result in favorable disease control has contributed to interest in investigating the feasibility of deintensification of the treatment of HPV-related OPSCC with multiple clinical trials that are currently recruiting patients.[51–54]

Surgical resection of oropharynx cancer can be curative when used as a single modality for patients with stage I to III tumors. Even patients with stage IV disease, who usually require adjuvant radiation or chemoradiation after resection, are likely to receive lower doses of radiation than would be needed in definitive radiotherapy treatment with curative intent, and concurrent chemotherapy

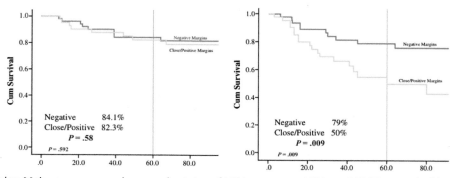

Fig. 4. Kaplan-Meier curve comparing margin status of HPV +ve versus HPV –ve OPSCC treated with primary surgery. (*From* Iyer NG, Dogan S, Palmer F, et al. Detailed analysis of clinicopathologic factors demonstrate distinct difference in outcome and prognostic factors between surgically treated HPV-positive and negative oropharyngeal cancer. Ann Surg Oncol 2015;22(13):4419; with permission.)

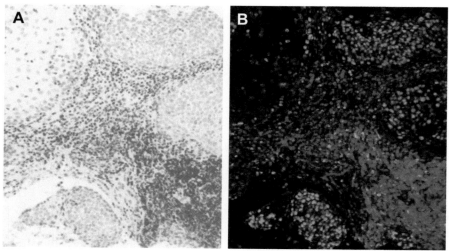

Fig. 5. (*A*) An HPV-positive OPSCC specimen (conventional hematoxylin-eosin, original magnification ×100). (*B*) Multispectral image of the same section showing immune infiltrate in TME (standard haematoxylin, original magnification ×100; Ki67 = *orange*; CD8 = *green*; PD-L1 = *red*; CD3 = *purple*).

might be avoided altogether. Surgical therapy allows more appropriate use of postoperative adjuvant therapy based on pathologic staging and has the potential to diminish substantially the need for high-dose radiation or concurrent chemoradiation in patients who are expected to do well.

FUTURE DIRECTIONS

The current standard of care for the evaluation of any surgical margin is with histopathological examination looking at the cellular morphology (mitotic figures, cytoplasm/nucleus ratio) and architecture (invasion into basement membrane, degree of differentiation). The use of these optical devices has been mainly studies to better delineate premalignant lesions from benign lesions. With regard to assessment of resection margins, the 2 more commonly used techniques, optical fluorescence imaging (OFI) and narrow band imaging (NBI), are capable of showing tissue changes at the microscopic and molecular levels.

Optical Fluorescence Imaging

OFI illuminates tissue with near-ultraviolet light. Fluorescence is the ability of certain molecules to absorb light at a particular wavelength and emit light of a longer wavelength (fluorophores). Within native tissue, this property is called autofluorescence. The fluorophores can be located in the tissue matrix or in cells (ie, collagen, elastin, keratin, and nicotinamide adenine dinucleotide hydride [NADH]). Dysplastic tissue or carcinoma has increased thickness of collagen and epithelium resulting in decreased fluorescence.[55] The epithelial layer shields the strongly

fluorescent collagen layer; therefore, the recorded fluorescence signal will be lower in the case of hyperplasia. In carcinoma, the increase in cell metabolism changes the balance between the fluorescent NADH (increase) and nonfluorescent NAD+ (decrease).[55]

Currently, clinical use of OFI has been mainly aimed at differentiating benign, dysplastic, and malignant lesions. There is limited study looking at OFI for the analysis of surgical margins. Francisco and colleagues[56] looked at the use of OFI in oral cavity carcinoma with comparison with normal mucosa. They found that OFI was able to discriminate between oral mucosa, injury, margins, and areas of recurrence using a homemade spectroscopy device at 406-nm wavelength without extrinsic fluorescent dyes.

Betz and colleagues[57] studied autofluorescence imaging in 30 patients with a tumor of the oral mucosa or oropharynx. They found sufficient to excellent demarcation by lower fluorescence intensity in 20 tumors. However, the tumors were not distinguishable from normal tissues. The tumors were all located on the tongue, soft palate, or the tonsillar sinus. They concluded that flat epithelial lesions were able to be subjectively better delineated by autofluorescence imaging than large, exophytic tumors. The investigators stated that porphyrinlike fluorescence is not a good diagnostic indicator. According to the investigators, the porphyrins are by-products of microbes and therefore limited to the necrotic surface of ulcerated tumors. Furthermore, only 33% of the tumors were mostly covered by strongly red fluorescing material. The observed red spots did not seem to spread homogeneously over the lesions surfaces, which made porphyrin fluorescence unsuitable for the demarcation of oral cancer.

The currently optical devices that are based on the use of OFI include VELscope (LED Dental, White Rock, British Columbia, Canada), ViziLite (Zila Pharmaceuticals, Phoenix, Arizona), ViziLite Plus with toluidine blue (Zila Pharmaceuticals), Microlux DL (AdDent, Danbury, Connecticut), Orascoptic DK (Orascoptic, a Kerr Company, Middleton, Wisconsin), and OralCDx (Oral CDx Laboratories, Suffern, New York).

Narrow Band Imaging

NBI (Olympus Medical Systems Corporation, Tokyo, Japan) is an endoscopic optical imaging enhancement technology that improves the contrast of the mucosal surface texture and submucosal vasculature. The use of NBI enables clinicians to identify premalignant and malignant lesions based on enhancement of the tumor angiogenesis and microvascular morphology. OPSCC has been addressed in 2 different case series. Tirelli and colleagues[58] examined equally distributed 26 patients who had oral and oropharynx SCC resection guided by NBI and compared the rate of positive margins at definitive histology with a historical cohort of 44 patients without the use of intraoperative NBI. They showed that the use of high-resolution microendoscopy imaging during TORS provided real-time histologic assessment of tumor margins with a statistically significant reduction in the rate of positive superficial margins at definitive histology. Tateya and colleagues[59] evaluated the feasibility and efficacy of NBI in determining the extent of OPSCC resection by TORS and found that it enabled an estimation of the horizontal extent of the superficial lesion and detection of surrounding superficial lesions normally not identified without NBI.

Intraoperative Ultrasound

Clayburgh and colleagues[60] attempted to address the absence of any haptic feedback when using TORS by using intraoperative imaging with real-time ultrasound to augment the 3-dimensional visualization of the robotic system. Ultrasound imaging was used for identification of the tumor boundary and the vascular structure within the tongue base and laryngopharyngeal wall, with the goal of improving the safety of oncologic resection and avoidance of major blood vessels. Through their case series of 10 patients, they were able to define the deep margin of a tongue-base tumor, thereby providing a guide for tumor resection. The ultrasound provided an accurate measurement of the tumor thickness when compared with the pathologic specimen, within 1 to 2 mm of the grossly measured tumor thickness. The use of intraoperative ultrasound allowed for focused, careful dissection to protect and avoid blood vessels during dissection as well as improved tumor resection.

Molecular Markers of Margins

With better understanding of oncogenesis, molecular markers have been used more frequently to help determine epigenetic changes within a clonal population of cells. The mechanism underlying these epigenetic changes include gene rearrangement, amplification, deletion, methylation and/or mutation.[61] It must be noted that targeted molecular margin analysis at present time is still evolving and not yet clinically practical. The approach of analyzing molecular margins addresses mucosal genetic alterations, before histomorphologic changes are evident. The implication of molecular analysis to guide the extent of surgery is yet to be determined; but at the present, the knowledge about these molecular markers is associated with response to chemoradiotherapy.

It is worth noting that in the era of immunotherapy for treatment of head and neck cancer, there is ongoing research to determine the markers that can be used to predict responders and nonresponders of immunotherapy. Analysis of gene expression profiles of tumors has identified a subgroup of patients with a particular gene expression pattern associated with immune responses. This subgroup has been termed an inflammatory TME. Tumors with an inflammatory TME demonstrate an upregulation of CD8$^+$–driven suppressive elements, such as regulatory T cells and programmed death ligand 1 (PD-L1). This inflamed phenotype has been shown to improve the activity of checkpoint blockers like anti–PD-1 or anti–PD-L1. Therefore, when considering the use of checkpoint inhibitors, one of the most actively researched area in immune-oncology is discovering a method to prime the antitumor response in the noninflamed phenotype.

There is good evidence to support that OPSCC associated with favorable outcomes differ by immune cell infiltrates; these differences are specific for tumor site and correlate with response to surgery, radiation, or chemotherapy.[62] This finding is further supported by Ward and colleagues,[63] who suggested that an immune response, reflected by TIL levels in the primary tumor, has an important role in the improved survival seen in most HPV-positive patients and is relevant for the clinical evaluation of HPV-positive OPSCC.

SUMMARY

If a margin is considered adequate, it is implied by this surgical definition that the resection encompasses all the cancerous cells. Unlike oral cavity SCC, whereby even with the best efforts at achieving clear margins there is still a 10% to 30% local recurrence rate. HPV-related OPSCC has lower locoregional recurrence rates despite close or positive margins. The impact of adjuvant chemoradiation in the setting of positive surgical margins remains unclear but is likely influenced by tumor biology. The favorable outcome may be contributed by a combination of the degree of surgical cytoreduction and the inflamed tumor microenvironment, thereby placing cytoreductive surgery as a viable surgical option to reduce tumor burden and decrease the burden of tumor-derived immunosuppression. It is feasible that surgical resection can be combined with immunotherapy to induce an effective immune response and overcome immunosuppression in the tumor microenvironment.[64] Future directions will allow for a reliable and more accurate assessment of margins on a molecular level to guide precise excision. In the meantime, whatever method is chosen for surgical management of OPSCC, there is a strong suggestion that in HPV-related OPSCC, narrow (<5 mm) or positive margins do not equate to higher locoregional recurrence or poorer survival.[48,65] Conversely, the prognosis of HPV negative or HPV positive with significant smoking history remains poor with high rates of locoregional recurrence. More robust clinical data are required for treatment strategies of HPV-negative OPSCC.

REFERENCES

1. Alicandri-Ciufelli M, Bonali M, Piccinini A, et al. Surgical margins in head and neck squamous cell carcinoma: what is 'close'? Eur Arch Otorhinolaryngol 2013;270:2603–9.
2. Siegel RL, Miller KD, Jemal A. Cancer statistics, 2015. CA Cancer J Clin 2015;65:5–29.
3. Hansson BG, Rosenquist K, Antonsson A, et al. Strong association between infection with human papillomavirus and oral and oropharyngeal squamous cell carcinoma: a population-based case-control study in southern Sweden. Acta Otolaryngol 2005;125:1337–44.
4. Mork J, Lie AK, Glattre E, et al. Human papillomavirus infection as a risk factor for squamous-cell carcinoma of the head and neck. N Engl J Med 2001; 344:1125–31.
5. Petrelli F, Sarti E, Barni S. Predictive value of human papillomavirus in oropharyngeal carcinoma treated with radiotherapy: an updated systematic review and meta-analysis of 30 trials. Head Neck 2014;36: 750–9.
6. O'Rorke MA, Ellison MV, Murray LJ, et al. Human papillomavirus related head and neck cancer survival: a systematic review and meta-analysis. Oral Oncol 2012;48:1191–201.
7. Huang SH, Xu W, Waldron J, et al. Refining American Joint Committee on Cancer/Union for International Cancer Control TNM stage and prognostic groups for human papillomavirus-related oropharyngeal carcinomas. J Clin Oncol 2015;33:836–45.
8. Ang KK, Harris J, Wheeler R, et al. Human papillomavirus and survival of patients with oropharyngeal cancer. N Engl J Med 2010;363:24–35.
9. Gillison ML, Chaturvedi AK, Anderson WF, et al. Epidemiology of human papillomavirus-positive head and neck squamous cell carcinoma. J Clin Oncol 2015;33:3235–42.
10. Chaturvedi AK, Engels EA, Pfeiffer RM, et al. Human papillomavirus and rising oropharyngeal cancer incidence in the United States. J Clin Oncol 2011; 29:4294–301.
11. Gooris PJ, Worthington P, Evans JR. Mandibulotomy: a surgical approach to oral and pharyngeal lesions. Int J Oral Maxillofac Surg 1989;18: 359–64.
12. Singh AM, Bahadur S, Tandon DA, et al. Anterior mandibulotomy for oral and oropharyngeal tumours. J Laryngol Otol 1993;107:316–9.
13. Selek U, Garden AS, Morrison WH, et al. Radiation therapy for early-stage carcinoma of the oropharynx. Int J Radiat Oncol Biol Phys 2004;59:743–51.
14. Cmelak AJ, Li S, Goldwasser MA, et al. Phase II trial of chemoradiation for organ preservation in resectable stage III or IV squamous cell carcinomas of the larynx or oropharynx: results of Eastern Cooperative Oncology Group Study E2399. J Clin Oncol 2007;25:3971–7.
15. Parsons JT, Mendenhall WM, Stringer SP, et al. Squamous cell carcinoma of the oropharynx: surgery, radiation therapy, or both. Cancer 2002;94: 2967–80.
16. Denis F, Garaud P, Bardet E, et al. Late toxicity results of the GORTEC 94-01 randomized trial comparing radiotherapy with concomitant radiochemotherapy for advanced-stage oropharynx carcinoma: comparison of LENT/SOMA, RTOG/EORTC, and NCI-CTC scoring systems. Int J Radiat Oncol Biol Phys 2003;55:93–8.
17. Shiley SG, Hargunani CA, Skoner JM, et al. Swallowing function after chemoradiation for advanced stage oropharyngeal cancer. Otolaryngol Head Neck Surg 2006;134:455–9.
18. Steiner W. Results of curative laser microsurgery of laryngeal carcinomas. Am J Otolaryngol 1993;14: 116–21.

19. Steiner W, Ambrosch G, Hess C, et al. Organ preservation by transoral laser microsurgery in piriform sinus carcinoma. Otolaryngol Head Neck Surg 2001;124:58–67.

20. Steiner W, Fierek O, Ambrosch P, et al. Transoral laser microsurgery for squamous cell carcinoma of the base of the tongue. Arch Otolaryngol Head Neck Surg 2003;129:36–43.

21. Haughey BH, Hinni ML, Salassa JR, et al. Transoral laser microsurgery as primary treatment for advanced-stage oropharyngeal cancer: a United States multicenter study. Head Neck 2011;33: 1683–94.

22. Williams CE, Kinshuck AJ, Derbyshire SG, et al. Transoral laser resection versus lip-split mandibulotomy in the management of oropharyngeal squamous cell carcinoma (OPSCC): a case match study. Eur Arch Otorhinolaryngol 2014; 271:367–72.

23. Weinstein GS, O'Malley BW, Snyder W, et al. Transoral robotic surgery: radical tonsillectomy. Arch Otolaryngol Head Neck Surg 2007;133:1220–6.

24. Park ES, Shum JW, Bui TG, et al. Robotic surgery: a new approach to tumors of the tongue base, oropharynx, and hypopharynx. Oral Maxillofac Surg Clin North Am 2013;25:49–59.

25. O'Malley BW, Weinstein GS, Snyder W, et al. Transoral robotic surgery (TORS) for base of tongue neoplasms. Laryngoscope 2006;116:1465–72.

26. Kumar B, Cordell KG, Lee JS, et al. EGFR, p16, HPV Titer, Bcl-xL and p53, sex, and smoking as indicators of response to therapy and survival in oropharyngeal cancer. J Clin Oncol 2008;26:3128–37.

27. Chung CH, Gillison ML. Human papillomavirus in head and neck cancer: its role in pathogenesis and clinical implications. Clin Cancer Res 2009;15: 6758–62.

28. Yu L, Wang L, Li M, et al. Expression of toll-like receptor 4 is down-regulated during progression of cervical neoplasia. Cancer Immunol Immunother 2010;59:1021–8.

29. Jouhi L, Datta N, Renkonen S, et al. Expression of toll-like receptors in HPV-positive and HPV-negative oropharyngeal squamous cell carcinoma–an in vivo and in vitro study. Tumour Biol 2015;36:7755–64.

30. Burdelya LG, Krivokrysenko VI, Tallant TC, et al. An agonist of toll-like receptor 5 has radioprotective activity in mouse and primate models. Science 2008; 320:226–30.

31. Kauppila JH, Mattila AE, Karttunen TJ, et al. Toll-like receptor 5 (TLR5) expression is a novel predictive marker for recurrence and survival in squamous cell carcinoma of the tongue. Br J Cancer 2013; 108:638–43.

32. Swick AD, Chatterjee A, De Costa AMA, et al. Modulation of therapeutic sensitivity by human papillomavirus. Radiother Oncol 2015;116:342–5.

33. Nordfors C, Grün N, Tertipis N, et al. CD8+ and CD4+ tumour infiltrating lymphocytes in relation to human papillomavirus status and clinical outcome in tonsillar and base of tongue squamous cell carcinoma. Eur J Cancer 2013;49:2522–30.

34. Badoual C, Hans S, Merillon N, et al. PD-1-expressing tumor-infiltrating T cells are a favorable prognostic biomarker in HPV-associated head and neck cancer. Cancer Res 2013;73:128–38.

35. Tertipis N, Villabona L, Nordfors C, et al. HLA-A* 02 in relation to outcome in human papillomavirus positive tonsillar and base of tongue cancer. Anticancer Res 2014;34:2369–75.

36. Turksma AW, Bontkes HJ, van den Heuvel H, et al. Effector memory T-cell frequencies in relation to tumour stage, location and HPV status in HNSCC patients. Oral Dis 2013;19:577–84.

37. Cohen MA, Weinstein GS, O'Malley BW, et al. Transoral robotic surgery and human papillomavirus status: oncologic results. Head Neck 2011;33: 573–80.

38. Karatzanis AD, Psychogios G, Waldfahrer F, et al. Surgical management of T1 oropharyngeal carcinoma. Head Neck 2012;34:1277–82.

39. Moore EJ, Henstrom DK, Olsen KD, et al. Transoral resection of tonsillar squamous cell carcinoma. Laryngoscope 2009;119:508–15.

40. Weinstein GS, O'Malley BW, Magnuson JS, et al. Transoral robotic surgery: a multicenter study to assess feasibility, safety, and surgical margins. Laryngoscope 2012;122:1701–7.

41. Ford SE, Brandwein-Gensler M, Carroll WR, et al. Transoral robotic versus open surgical approaches to oropharyngeal squamous cell carcinoma by human papillomavirus status. Otolaryngol Head Neck Surg 2014;151:606–11.

42. de Almeida JR, Li R, Magnuson JS, et al. Oncologic outcomes after transoral robotic surgery: a multi-institutional study. JAMA Otolaryngol Head Neck Surg 2015;141:1043–51.

43. Kwok P, Gleich O, Hübner G, et al. Prognostic importance of clear versus revised margins in oral and pharyngeal cancer. Head Neck 2010;32: 1479–84.

44. Patel RS, Goldstein DP, Guillemaud J, et al. Impact of positive frozen section microscopic tumor cut-through revised to negative on oral carcinoma control and survival rates. Head Neck 2010;32:1444–51.

45. Meier JD, Oliver DA, Varvares MA. Surgical margin determination in head and neck oncology: current clinical practice. The results of an International American Head and Neck Society Member Survey. Head Neck 2005;27:952–8.

46. Grant DG, Salassa JR, Hinni ML, et al. Carcinoma of the tongue base treated by transoral laser microsurgery, part two: persistent, recurrent and second primary tumors. Laryngoscope 2006;116:2156–61.

47. Weinstein GS, Quon H, Newman HJ, et al. Transoral robotic surgery alone for oropharyngeal cancer: an analysis of local control. Arch Otolaryngol Head Neck Surg 2012;138:628–34.

48. Iyer NG, Dogan S, Palmer F, et al. Detailed analysis of clinicopathologic factors demonstrate distinct difference in outcome and prognostic factors between surgically treated HPV-positive and negative oropharyngeal cancer. Ann Surg Oncol 2015;22: 4411–21.

49. Sload R, Silver N, Jawad BA, et al. The role of transoral robotic surgery in the management of HPV negative oropharyngeal squamous cell carcinoma. Curr Oncol Rep 2016;18:53.

50. Urban D, Corry J, Rischin D. What is the best treatment for patients with human papillomavirus-positive and -negative oropharyngeal cancer? Cancer 2014; 120:1462–70.

51. Transoral surgery followed by low-dose or standard-dose radiation therapy with or without chemotherapy in treating patients with HPV positive stage III-IVA oropharyngeal cancer. ClinicalTrials.gov. Available at: https://www.clinicaltrials.gov/ct2/show/NCT01898494 #sthash.fVUj9pyq.dpuf. Accessed June 11, 2016.

52. Reduced-dose intensity-modulated radiation therapy with or without cisplatin in treating patients with advanced oropharyngeal cancer. ClinicalTrials. gov. Available at: https://www.clinicaltrials.gov/ct2/ show/NCT02254278#sthash.fVUj9pyq.dpuf. Accessed June 11, 2016.

53. The quarterback trial: reduced dose radiotherapy for HPV+ oropharynx cancer. Full text view. Available at: https://clinicaltrials.gov/ct2/show/NCT0 1706939. Accessed June 11, 2016.

54. Owadally W, Hurt C, Timmins H, et al. PATHOS: a phase II/III trial of risk-stratified, reduced intensity adjuvant treatment in patients undergoing transoral surgery for human papillomavirus (HPV) positive oropharyngeal cancer. BMC Cancer 2015;15:602.

55. De Veld DCG, Witjes MJH, Sterenborg HJCM, et al. The status of in vivo autofluorescence spectroscopy and imaging for oral oncology. Oral Oncol 2005;41: 117–31.

56. Francisco AL, Correr WR, Pinto CA, et al. Analysis of surgical margins in oral cancer using in situ fluorescence spectroscopy. Oral Oncol 2014;50:593–9.

57. Betz CS, Mehlmann M, Rick K, et al. Autofluorescence imaging and spectroscopy of normal and malignant mucosa in patients with head and neck cancer. Lasers Surg Med 1999;25:323–34.

58. Tirelli G, Piovesana M, Gatto A, et al. Is NBI-guided resection a breakthrough for achieving adequate resection margins in oral and oropharyngeal squamous cell carcinoma? Ann Otol Rhinol Laryngol 2016;125:596–601.

59. Tateya I, Ishikawa S, Morita S, et al. Magnifying endoscopy with narrow band imaging to determine the extent of resection in transoral robotic surgery of oropharyngeal cancer. Case Rep Otolaryngol 2014;2014:604737.

60. Clayburgh DR, Byrd JK, Bonfili J, et al. Intraoperative ultrasonography during transoral robotic surgery. Ann Otol Rhinol Laryngol 2016; 125:37–42.

61. Lingen MW, Pinto A, Mendes RA, et al. Genetics/epigenetics of oral premalignancy: current status and future research. Oral Dis 2011;17(Suppl 1):7–22.

62. Wansom D, Light E, Thomas D, et al. Infiltrating lymphocytes and human papillomavirus-16–associated oropharyngeal cancer. Laryngoscope 2012;122: 121–7.

63. Ward MJ, Thirdborough SM, Mellows T, et al. Tumour-infiltrating lymphocytes predict for outcome in HPV-positive oropharyngeal cancer. Br J Cancer 2014;110:489–500.

64. Bell RB, Gough MJ, Seung SK, et al. Cytoreductive surgery for head and neck squamous cell carcinoma in the new age of immunotherapy. Oral Oncol 2016;61:166–76.

65. Kaczmar JM, Tan KS, Heitjan DF, et al. HPV-related oropharyngeal cancer: risk factors for treatment failure in patients managed with primary transoral robotic surgery. Head Neck 2016;38:59–65.

Evaluation of the Bone Margin in Oral Squamous Cell Carcinoma

Joshua E. Lubek, DDS, MD*, Kelly R. Magliocca, DDS, MPH

KEYWORDS

- Marginal mandibulectomy • Segmental mandibulectomy • Bone invasion
- Squamous cell carcinoma

KEY POINTS

- The infiltrative pattern of bone invasion has a higher risk of local recurrence and lower disease-specific survival.
- Bone invasion at the dentoalveolar-tooth bearing segment does not pathologically upstage a tumor (pTNM staging).
- Marginal mandibulectomy is an oncologically safe procedure in select patients without compromising esthetic or functional outcomes.
- At least 1 cm of inferior border is required to prevent pathologic fracture after marginal mandibulectomy.
- Intraoperative bone marrow assessment can be a valuable tool providing for a real-time analysis of medullary bone invasion.

PATTERNS OF BONE INVASION AND SPREAD

Previous belief was that oral cavity lymphatics passed through the mandible en route to cervical lymphatics. It was not until Marchetta and colleagues[1] established that oral squamous cell carcinoma invades the mandible by direct extension and not via lymphatic periosteal channels. This finding has been validated by more recent investigations and has led to the ability for the possibility of more conservative marginal resection with preservation of function and cosmesis.[2] Despite this development, the ability to identify those tumors with bone invasion that will affect prognosis and require more aggressive treatment is still difficult.

Current literature would suggest that it is not necessarily bone invasion that affects prognosis, but rather the pattern of bone invasion as initially described by Slootweg and Muller.[3] In the less aggressive "erosive" pattern, the tumor invades on a broad front, eroding the bone directly adjacent to it. Tumors of this pattern do not invade the periodontal ligament or inferior alveolar nerve (IAN) canal. The "infiltrative" pattern presents histologically as fingers or islands of tumor invading the cancellous marrow space without intervening connective tissue and with few osteoclasts visualized. This aggressive pattern is highly destructive invading the IAN canal with resultant perineural invasion[4] (**Fig. 1**). In a series by Shaw and colleagues,[5] patients who were found to have an "infiltrative" pattern of spread had significantly higher rates of local recurrence (40% vs 16%) and 5-year disease-specific survival (43% vs 76%) as compared with the "erosive" pattern, respectively. Interestingly, the authors found no statistical difference in local recurrence or disease specific survival when comparing patients with the "erosive" pattern with those patients who did not have any bony involvement histologically. In a series by

Oral-Head & Neck Surgery/Microvascular Surgery, Department of Oral & Maxillofacial Surgery, University of Maryland, 650 West Baltimore Street, Room 1215, Baltimore, MD 21201, USA
* Corresponding author.
E-mail address: jlubek@umaryland.edu

Oral Maxillofacial Surg Clin N Am 29 (2017) 281–292
http://dx.doi.org/10.1016/j.coms.2017.03.005

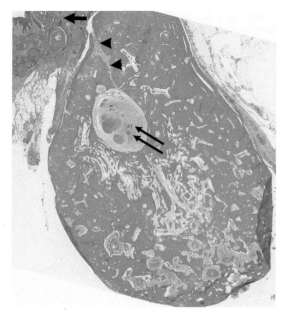

Fig. 1. Cross section of squamous cell carcinoma (SCCa) of alveolar ridge and buccal vestibule, hematoxylin & eosin (H&E) staining, scanning magnification. Primary site SCCa (*thick black arrow*), infiltrates into mandible via bone clefts (*arrow heads*), to permeate within inferior alveolar canal (*thin arrows*) and mandibular marrow space.

O'Brien and colleagues,[6] of the 127 patients who underwent marginal and segmental resection local control, survival was not significantly negatively affected by bone invasion but rather only a positive soft tissue margin. The authors, however, did not specify the histologic pattern of bone invasion within the mandible.

The general route of bone invasion in the dentate patient is thought to be via the overlying gingival mucosa with entry into the periodontal ligament toward the apex of the socket and ultimately into the marrow. Marrow invasion in the edentulous patient can occur in areas of cortical bone defects at previous extraction sites or bony vascular channels.[5,7]

The attached gingiva overlying the alveolar bone is approximately 2 to 3 mm in thickness and susceptible to early bone invasion. Because the alveolar bone is generally thin and without significant marrow component the question arises as to what is the significance of this bone invasion at the alveolar region. Gomez and colleagues[8] reported on a series of 83 gingival tumors, and found that bone invasion is an early event and not necessarily an indication of advanced/aggressive disease. Until recently, there was no differentiation in the TNM staging of bone invasion involving this subsite, resulting in all tumors being upstaged to T4a status. Recent guidelines have suggested that superficial/alveolar bone invasion does not result in T4a upstaging because there is inconclusive evidence as to worse prognosis with such alveolar bone involvement.[9,10] A recent large retrospective series of 345 mandibular gingival squamous cell carcinoma reported that medullary bone invasion was pathologically identified in only 53% of patients (107/201) with clinical invasion through cortical bone on imaging. The authors concluded that medullary bone involvement is not only insufficient for T4a staging, but only medullary involvement of the IAN canal actually impacted overall survival. Interestingly, the study reported that medullary involvement was associated with risk of distant disease.[11]

PREDICTORS OF MAXILLARY AND MANDIBULAR BONE INVOLVEMENT

In the absence of obvious clinical factors such as gross tumor with tooth mobility, pathologic fracture, or significant bone loss on imaging, the preoperative assessment of bone invasion becomes a more difficult task. Ultimately, the goal is to improve oncologic surgical safety while minimizing patient morbidity. At the current time, there is no specific single test that will provide the surgeon with 100% accuracy the ability to predict which patient can undergo marginal versus segmental resection. However, with a thorough clinical and radiologic imaging examination, in conjunction with an understanding of tumor characteristics, an accurate preoperative assessment can greatly improve outcomes.

Pandey and colleagues[12] reported on a prospective series of 51 patients undergoing segmental mandibular resection in an attempt to identify risk factors that would help to predict mandibular invasion. The authors concluded that lesions within 1 cm of the mandible (with or without mandibular fixation), poorly differentiated tumors, sensory disturbances of the IAN, and cortical expansion significantly increased the odds risk ratio for mandibular bone invasion.

Previous dental extraction can become a source of great confusion in the assessment of bone invasion. In most scenarios, a biopsy has been performed either simultaneously with tooth extraction or after treatment of a longstanding, nonhealing extraction socket. The treating oncologic surgeon is now left to ponder if there was gross mobility before treatment, bone graft material placed, or has the socket been aggressively curetted thus seeding tumor cells into the marrow space? Imaging becomes more difficult owing to bone loss secondary to extraction or remodeling and inflammation (ie, false-positive computed tomography [CT] scan/MRI or PET scan, respectively). In a published retrospective series by the current author, 17 of 72 patients with squamous cell carcinoma of the gingiva underwent previous dental extraction. The authors concluded that patients had been clinically upstaged and that dental extraction did not increase risk of nodal spread or act as a marker of worse prognosis. On survival analysis, bony invasion did not correlate with a worse outcome.[13] In a series of mandibular gingival squamous cell carcinoma by Overholt and colleagues,[14] 28 patients had undergone a dental extraction, in which the authors did not find any statistical significant effect on local recurrence or overall survival. Unfortunately, the authors do not differentiate between those patients who underwent marginal versus segmental mandibulectomy and those who received dental extraction. A possible explanation for this similar outcome could be that those patients with previous extractions underwent a larger, more comprehensive operation (ie, segmental mandibulectomy). Yamagata and colleagues[15] compared a cohort of 19 patients (13 nonextractions and 6 extractions) who underwent treatment for gingival carcinoma. Bone invasion was identified in all patients with previous dental extraction and in 68% of those patients who did not have dental extractions. The overall survival for mandibular squamous cell carcinoma was 84.6% versus 65.8% respectively (worse in the extraction group); however, this did not attain statistical significance. Interestingly, patients with maxillary gingival squamous cell carcinoma who had previous extractions had a worse prognosis. The authors suggest that the less dense cortical bone within the maxilla allows for ease of access to the marrow space and advocate aggressive surgical resection. Shingaki and colleagues[16] did not find any outcomes difference in their reported series of 47 patients with bone invasion who underwent previous dental extraction before treatment of a mandibular gingival squamous cell carcinoma.

Previous radiation is thought to impact periosteal vascularity, thus decreasing the ability of the periosteum to act as a barrier preventing tumor invasion and spread. McGregor and MacDonald[17] evaluated 16 irradiated mandibles identifying that routes of entry were both more variable and with multiple foci noting breakdown within the periosteum as compared with mandibular bone invasion patterns in nonirradiated bone. Despite this finding, there are lacking data as to the true effect of radiation and increased risk of bone invasion. In the series by Pandey and colleagues,[12] a total of 23 recurrent cancers had received prior radiotherapy, were not found to be at higher risk of mandibular bone invasion as compared with 28 patients never having received irradiation. Contrary to the previously mentioned series, Namin and colleagues[18] reported on a series of 51 patients undergoing mandibular resection and concluded that patients with prior radiation did have a significantly higher incidence in bone invasion compared with nonradiated patients.

Perineural invasion is generally a predictor of poor prognosis and increased local recurrence however few studies look at symptomatic sensory disturbances of the IAN and bone invasion. One would logically assume that, if the nerve is involved, direct extension through the cancellous bone and into the nerve canal must have occurred. Pandey and colleagues[12] reported that on univariate analysis IAN sensory disturbances predicted for bone invasion; however, this was not an independent predictor because it was not statistically significant on multivariate analysis. Sanchis and colleagues[19] reported on mental neuropathy secondary to squamous carcinoma with a mean overall survival rate of 28 months.

IMAGING TECHNIQUES

Preoperative imaging is an invaluable tool to aid in the assessment of bone marrow invasion. Controversy still exists as to which imaging will yield the most accurate results while minimizing financial costs. Various imaging modalities have been studied and the most common techniques, which include orthopantomogram, CT imaging, MRI, PET, and single photon emission computed tomography (SPECT) scans, will be detailed.

Orthopantomogram is an inexpensive technique that can provide an excellent view of the mandibular body, ramus, and inferior alveolar bony canal. Limitations include spine artifact that can obscure a detailed view of the symphyseal region, and differentiation between periodontal disease and erosion secondary to tumor. Orthopantomogram is regarded as a low sensitivity test owing to the fact that at least 30% to 50% cortical bone demineralization must occur for visible change on radiographic imaging. It is a useful image that should be used in conjunction with other imaging modalities.[20] In a series of 67 patients, Acton and colleagues[21] reported that orthopantomogram alone had a sensitivity, specificity, and positive/negative predictive value of 80%, 72%, 75%, and 77%, respectively (**Fig. 2**A).

CT scan and MRI are the most common modalities used in the assessment of bone invasion. They are generally considered first-line imaging, providing clinical information of extent of bone involvement, the surrounding soft tissue infiltrated, and cervical metastases. CT scan offers the advantage of lower cost and faster operating times, especially beneficial in patients who cannot remain still for prolonged periods or have significant anxiety

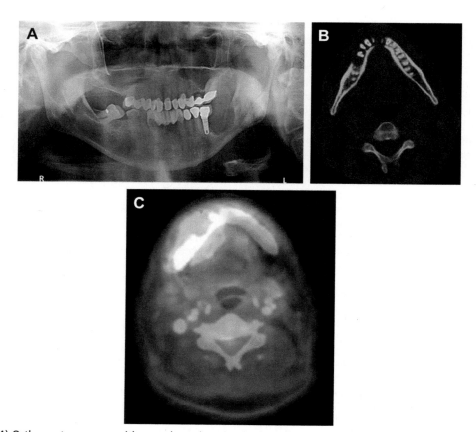

Fig. 2. (A) Orthopantomogram with gross bone invasion in the left posterior mandible associated with a dental endosseous implant. (B) Mandibular bone destruction with medullary invasion identified on high resolution computed tomography scan. (C) Medullary bone invasion as identified on PET/computed tomography fusion imaging.

or claustrophobia. Higher resolution CT scans can also allow for very fine sliced images (1 mm), further enhancing bone detail. MRI avoids the use of radiation but can overestimate the extent of bone invasion, especially in the face of significant edema or inflammation. Both types of modalities can be affected by dental artifact in patients' with heavily restored dentition. CT scan has a higher specificity for identifying bone invasion as compared with MRI, although MRI provides for better resolution of the marrow and involvement of the IAN with higher sensitivity. In a metaanalysis review, Brown and Lewis-Jones[22] reported an overall sensitivity and specificity of 75% and 86% versus 85% and 72% for CT scan and MRI, respectively. Interestingly, in a study by Van Cann and colleagues,[23] the authors reported very high specificity for both CT scan and MRI (95.7%-100%) with poor sensitivity for both imaging modalities (58.1%-62.8%). MRI has also been shown to have excellent sensitivity and negative predictive value in the evaluation of bone involvement within the maxilla.[24]

Cone beam CT scanning offers the advantages of low radiation dose, decreased interference with metal artifact, and low cost as compared with a conventional CT scan. It is reported to be highly accurate in the prediction of bone invasion with adjacent gingival squamous cell carcinoma. In a study by Brockenbrough and colleagues,[25] the cone beam CT scan accurately predicted mandibular invasion in 21 of 22 patients. In a recent large series of 197 patients with oral squamous cell carcinoma, cone beam CT scan was compared against bone scan and CT or MRI with comparable accuracy of 84.8% compared with 89.3% and 83.2%, respectively. Bone invasion was confirmed on histopathology and although bone scan was demonstrated to have a slightly higher level of accuracy it was statistically ($P = .188$) not significant.[26] Drawbacks to the cone beam CT scan include loss of image resolution with patient movement, difficulty in differentiation between tumor invasion and cortical irregularities, and the failure for soft tissue visualization necessitating either contrast-enhanced CT scan or MRI (**Fig. 2**B).

PET imaging to identify bone invasion is difficult owing to loss of spatial resolution secondary to "partial volume effect" that causes 3-dimensional blurring and spillover resulting in a signal that seems to be emanating from outside the actual tumor region.[27] Second, significant inflammation as in the case of a large tumor with an extensive soft tissue component, recent extraction, or periodontal disease can result in both false-negative and false-positive results. The combination of fused imaging with PET/CT or PET/MRI can have the advantage of providing accurate anatomic detail with metabolic tumor activity. Various studies have differed in results and efficacy of PET/CT in the delineation of oral squamous cell carcinoma bone invasion.[28,29] Babin and colleagues[29] reported 100% sensitivity with PET/CT scan for assessing bone invasion as compared with CT alone. Huang and colleagues[24] reported a lower sensitivity (80% in maxillary bone and 87.5% in the mandibular bone). Interestingly, in the previous series, the authors also compared the use of PET/MRI with a reported sensitivity of 100% as compared with PET/CT or CT alone. Their study also reported a greater sensitivity for assessing mandibular bone invasion as compared with MRI alone, but equivalent in the evaluation of maxillary bone invasion by carcinoma. The most common tracer used in PET imaging involves a tagged glucose (fluorine-18-fluorodeoxyglucose [18F-FDG]). The theory behind this involves the increased glucose uptake by hypermetabolic tumor cells. As described previously, both inflammation and spillover can result in false-positive activity. Recently, an amino acid tracer L-3-[(18) F]-fluoro-α-methyl tyrosine [(18)F-FAMT] that specifically is transported into cancer cells by L-type amino acid transporter 1 has been used in PET/CT imaging. L-type amino acid transporter 1 over-expression in tumors is correlated significantly with cell proliferation and angiogenesis. In a series by Kim and colleagues,[30] 27 patients with squamous carcinoma of the alveolar ridges were studied preoperatively for bone marrow invasion, using (18)F-FAMT PET/CT, (18)F-FDG PET/CT, and MRI. Results of the study demonstrated that (18)F-FAMT PET/CT was useful and more specific than MRI or (18)F-FDG PET/CT in the detection of bone marrow invasion of oral squamous cell carcinoma and may help to minimize the extent of surgical resection required (**Fig. 2**C).

Although not commonly used, bone scan imaging (SPECT) is considered to be useful in the detection of early bone invasion because bone mineral loss occurs earlier as compared with conventional imaging. In a series of 50 patients with bone invasion, SPECT was positive in all patients with pathologic bone invasion.[31] False-positive rates are reported to be as high as 40% with increased specificity in patients who do not have teeth within the vicinity of the tumor. Reasons suggested for false-positive rates include infection, soft tissue tumor inflammation, radiation osteonecrosis, and dental infections. Because a SPECT scan is considered highly specific, a negative SPECT scan can be used to rule out medullary bone invasion.

MARGINAL VERSUS SEGMENTAL RESECTION
Rim or Sagittal Resection

In the face of limited mandibular bone involvement, numerous studies have demonstrated that the marginal mandibular resection and the lingual sagittal rim mandibulectomy areoncologically safe procedures while providing decreased patient functional and esthetic morbidity.[2,32–35] Advantages include preservation of the IAN (sensory lip function), decreased operative times, and obviating the need for bone reconstruction often with microvascular free tissue transfer (ie, fibula or Deep circumflex iliac artery flap [DCIA]) or secondary bone grafting. Ultimately, the decision as to whether a segmental or marginal/rim resection will be performed depends on both oncologic and reconstructive factors during the clinical decision algorithm. From an oncologic viewpoint, medullary bone invasion or the inability to remove a large tumor without margin safety mandates a segmental bone resection. Reconstructive considerations include the risk of mandibular fracture as a result of reduced bone height or thickness, risk of osteoradionecrosis and compromised mandibular vascularity or anticipation of inadequate bone height for dental rehabilitation.

The marginal mandibulectomy removes the alveolar bone and associated teeth while preserving the IAN and basal bone keeping the inferior border of the mandible intact. The lingual sagittal rim mandibulectomy involves removal of the inner cortex of the mandible assuming that the adjacent tumor on the lingual aspect erodes through periosteum and the inner cortex is the lateral margin. In 1987, Barttelbort and Ariyan described the marginal mandibulectomy for management of floor of mouth squamous cell carcinoma with early bone invasion.[32] The authors found that it was an effective operation with local control rates comparable to those receiving a segmental resection. The authors, however, noted that approximately 15% of patients developed a mandibular fracture. In a follow-up study in 1993, the authors directly compared both types of mandibular preservation techniques (marginal mandibular resection/rim mandibulectomy) and the amount of bone required to resist fracture development.[36] The authors performed incremental osteotomies on fresh cadaver mandibles. Incremental weights were applied with strain gauges to measure load. Conclusions drawn from this study noted that the marginal mandibulectomy was superior to the lingual sagittal rim mandibulectomy in prevention of fracture and that ideally at least 1 cm of bone should remain at the inferior border to decrease the risk of postoperative fracture. Fractures were also more likely to happen at the vertical line angle osteotomy of the marginal resection. Based on these data many, clinicians will round the sharp osteotomy line angle and reinforce the remaining mandible with a reconstruction bar if there is less than 1 cm of native bone remaining at the inferior border (**Figs. 3**, **4A–C** and **5**).

Does marginal resection affect outcome in the face of bone invasion identified on postoperative pathology?

A significant dilemma arises when a marginal resection is performed and the final pathology reports a positive bone margin or invasion into the deep medullary bone. In an ideal situation, the surgeon would like to return to the operating room to convert the surgery into a segmental resection of the involved bone. This can prove to be quite difficult owing to extensive inflammation from recent surgery and the possibility of an overlying soft tissue flap in the preexisting surgical site. This is further compounded with the added morbidity of the need for a bone flap reconstruction. In a series by Chen and colleagues,[2] 43 patients underwent marginal mandibulectomy with 16% of patients having bone involvement on histopathologic examination. Surgical margins were negative at time of initial resection. In this series, 1 patient developed local recurrence that was noted to have soft tissue involvement as well. The authors concluded that

histologic evidence of bone invasion did not translate into a significant difference in local tumor control, bone recurrence rate, or 5-year disease-specific survival. The authors also mention that the incidence of osteoradionecrosis after marginal mandibulectomy and adjuvant radiotherapy was 17.4% (4 of 23 patients); however, mandibular bone invasion did not increase the risk of development of osteoradionecrosis.

Petrovic and colleagues[35] report on a recent series involving 326 patients who underwent a marginal mandibulectomy for early stage squamous cell carcinoma (T1/T2). Microscopic bone invasion was identified in 49 patients with medullary bone invasion in 13 of those subjects. The authors noted that 16% of patients had positive bone margins on final pathology. Interestingly, the authors reported that local recurrence-free survival was similar in patients with microscopic positive margins as long as adjuvant radiotherapy was delivered.

CLINICAL AND HISTOPATHOLOGIC INTRAOPERATIVE EVALUATION OF THE BONE MARGIN

When oral squamous cell carcinoma necessitates removal of bone, the position and placement of bone margins must be considered. The ideal oncologic surgical resection will remove disease, achieve negative bone margin (5 mm of resected bone free margin on histopathologic evaluation), and allow for appropriate reconstructive planning preoperatively (**Fig. 6**). Although a 5-mm margin of histopathologically uninvolved tissue surrounding the resected squamous cell carcinoma is most commonly accepted as a negative margin, the 'margin tissue' that is most often studied is composed of mucosa and/or soft tissue. There has been considerably less clinicopathologic study of the ideal measurement for a tumor-free bone margin.[17] Mucosa and soft tissue undergo variable shrinkage once removed from the patient but, given the rigidity of bone, this is less likely of

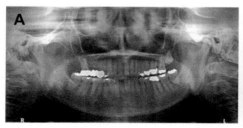
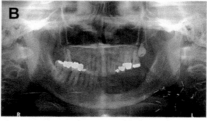

Fig. 3. (*A*) Orthopantomogram of a left posterior mandibular gingival squamous cell carcinoma. Bone invasion is not identified on imaging. The patient is planned for a marginal mandibulectomy. (*B*) Postoperative image orthopantomogram after marginal mandibulectomy for an early stage gingival squamous cell carcinoma.

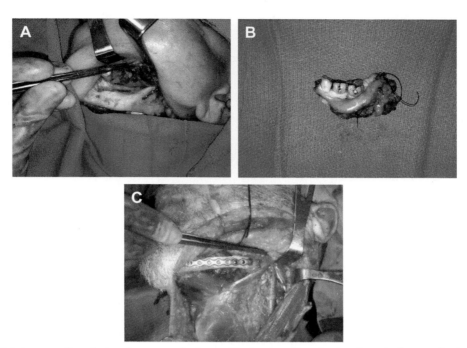

Fig. 4. (*A*) Intraoperative design for a marginal mandibular resection for treatment of an early stage gingivobuccal squamous cell carcinoma without cortical bone invasion. Bone margin is outlined in blue. (*B*) Marginal mandibulectomy pathologic specimen. Silk sutures are placed to orient and mark out the soft tissue margins for the pathologist. (*C*) Marginal mandibulectomy with minimal bone height and width remaining at the inferior border of the mandible. Mandibular reconstruction bar placed to help prevent pathologic fracture.

concern when planning the placement of clinical resection margins in bone. On balance, the precise position of the tumor within bone may be unclear, which could create ambiguity for the clinical placement of bone margins. Factors such as clinical inspection and imaging findings including panoramic radiograph, and CT scan may underestimate the width of invasive disease by 5 mm, 13 mm, and 5 mm respectively.[37] In 1988, McGregor and MacDonald[17] recommended planning a clinical resection of 0.5 to 1.0 cm of unaffected bone around the tumor and, more recently, 3 separate groups—Namin and colleagues,[18] Wysluch and colleagues,[38] and Weitz and colleagues[39]—report resection of at least 1.0 cm of uninvolved bone, as measured from either macroscopic tumor or suspected bone involvement. To achieve negative bone margins, the surgeon removes at least 1 tooth on either side of the tumor in a dentate patient, include

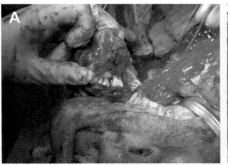
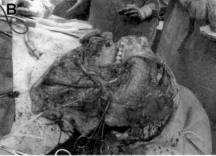

Fig. 5. (*A*) Segmental mandibular resection for an extensive squamous cell carcinoma with medullary bone involvement. Access via a lip-split incision. (*B*) Segmental mandibular composite resection defect with combined modified radical neck dissection.

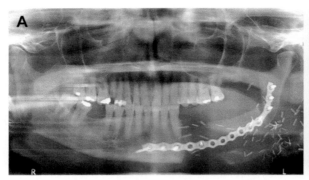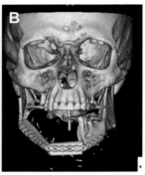

Fig. 6. (*A*) Orthopantomogram of a segmental mandibular defect reconstructed with a vascularized scapula osteocutaneous flap. (*B*) Three-dimensional computed tomography reconstruction imaging of a segmental mandibular defect reconstructed with a vascularized fibula osteocutaneous flap.

the entire nerve-bearing segment when marrow invasion is present or formal maxillectomy in cases of maxillary involvement. When the bone marrow is uninvolved by tumor, an oncologically safe marginal resection can often be performed. As described previously, this technique allows for preservation of mandibular continuity or low-level maxillectomy/alveolectomy with decreased reconstructive functional and cosmetic morbidity. At the current time, unless there is obvious marrow invasion as indicated on clinical preoperative examination (ie, gross visualization of tumor and tooth mobility) or imaging as described previously (loss of marrow signal, significant cortical bone loss on CT imaging/panorex, or invasion or pathologic fracture), the evaluation for possible bone invasion will be conducted intraoperatively by the surgeon, which also has limitations. Often the surgeon relies on a "peek and shriek" periosteal stripping technique visualizing tumor invasion through the periosteum and cortex. Even direct clinical evaluation can be difficult in situations involving previous radiation, prior/recent dental extraction, or dental infection. In a review of 35 patients with oral cavity squamous cell carcinoma, Brown and colleagues[37] found that periosteal stripping provided for an accurate real-time predictor of mandibular bone invasion (only 1 patient with a false-positive result). The authors concluded that marginal resection was safe and only if a positive periosteal intraoperative finding was identified should conversion to segmental resection be performed.

Limitations in methods to assess the pathologic status of a bone margin at the time of surgery can negatively affect prognosis. Guerra and colleagues[34] reported on a retrospective review of 106 patients who underwent either segmental or marginal mandibular resection. Those who were found to have tumor infiltration

beyond the resection margin had a statistical association with poor survival. The ability to return to the operative setting to revise a positive margin is also difficult because reconstruction is likely to have been performed. Revision of a bone margin involved by carcinoma has the potential to increase morbidity, may influence the postoperative plan for adjuvant therapy, and/or delay to adjuvant therapy, negatively affecting prognosis.

Intraoperative evaluation of bone and bone margins may provide critical information in key surgical decisions, such as detection of clinically occult bone invasion along the resection margin of a marginal mandibulectomy and/or assessing the adequacy surgical bone margins of a segmental mandibulectomy specimen. Intraoperative histologic evaluation of a complete cross-section of the cortical and medullary bone margin by conventional frozen section analysis is presently not possible in routine practice, owing to the need for decalcification procedures before sectioning of the bone. Therefore, investigators have most commonly reported on the assessment of intraoperative bone margin using 1 or 2 general approaches in clinical practice; the use of cytopathologic techniques and/or intraoperative histologic analysis of select portions of the bony margin using conventional frozen section. Direct comparison of these studies and techniques is limited by methodologic differences, the nature of the disease studied (predominantly, but not exclusively, squamous cell carcinoma), the type of surgical procedure performed, and location of the sampled bone margin.[18,38–44] Mahmood and colleagues[40] used intraoperative mandibular bone marrow cytologic scrapings to predict bone margin status that perfectly correlated with the final pathologic evaluation of the bone margins after decalcification in a group of 7 patients undergoing segmental resection of the mandible involved by squamous cell carcinoma. In 2015, Namin and colleagues,[18] described their experience with intraoperative bone marrow cytologic smears obtained from the specimen margin of marginal and/or segmental resections performed for squamous cell carcinoma. Six of 51 patients were identified with a positive bone marrow preparation intraoperatively, which led to additional bone resection in 1-cm increments and, subsequently, negative final bone margins. Accuracy of the technique was 100%, when compared with the gold standard histologic examination of the decalcified specimen bone margin. The authors also found that patients with initially positive bone margins did not have an adverse prognosis as compared with those with initially negative bone margins intraoperatively. In a cohort of 102 patients, Nieberer and colleagues[41] evaluated mandibular or maxillary bone margins during resection of squamous cell carcinoma with cytologic assessment intraoperatively, and reported a sensitivity and specificity of 94% and 97% respectively.

Other groups have evaluated histologic samples of bone and/or portions of the mandibular nerve intraoperatively with standard frozen section techniques to provide information on the adequacy of the bone resection. In a series of 30 patients, Forrest and colleagues[42] curetted and evaluated approximately 1 cm of cancellous bone obtained from the 'mandibular stump' remaining after resection of the mandible. Examination by standard frozen section technique predicted final bone margins with 97% accuracy when compared with the true bone margins obtained from conventional histologic sections of the formalin-fixed, decalcified resection specimen. Histologic sampling of cortical bone during routine frozen section analysis is nearly precluded by its dense mineralization, which hinders sectioning of the sample. Oxford and Ducic[43] described a technique using sharpened osteotomes of 4 to 5 mm thickness to obtain cortical bone specimens so thin as to obviate decalcification and permit evaluation using frozen section technique. In their series, the authors report a sensitivity and specificity of 89% and 100%, respectively, when correlating with final bone margins.[43]

In 2011, Bilodeau and Chiosea reviewed their institutional experience with intraoperative histologic evaluation of bone marrow curettings and/or IAN biopsies as a surrogate for bone margin status.[44] In 27 cases of segmental mandibular resection, 35 bone marrow specimens were evaluated, then later correlated with complete cross-sections of the formalin-fixed, decalcified bone margins. In this series, 6 true-positive bone margins and 3 false-negative intraoperative reports were identified, leading to a reported sensitivity and specificity of 50% and 100%, respectively. Sensitivity in this study may have been limited by sampling of the remaining mandibular osseous tissue within the tumor bed, rather than sampling of the resection specimen margins. Once perineural invasion of the intraosseous IAN has occurred, perineural spread of tumor could potentially be identified, and a possible surrogate for surgical bone margin compromise. In the recent prospective study by Weitz and colleagues[39] frozen section analysis of the IAN at the bone margin was evaluated as a surrogate for bone margin control. In 2 of 27 cases, the intraosseous neural stump at the specimen bone margin could not be identified. In the remaining 25 cases, neural specimens evaluated at frozen section and were deemed negative for squamous cell carcinoma. In 3 of 25 cases, atypical cells were identified during the frozen section evaluation, but were felt to be insufficient histologic evidence to support an intraoperative diagnosis of squamous cell carcinoma. In all 3 cases, however, positive bone margins were confirmed upon decalcification and further processing, leading the authors to estimate a sensitivity of 67% when 'atypical cells' were considered a clinically useful finding, but insensitive (sensitivity of 0%) in identifying invasive squamous cell carcinoma. In this study, extensive involvement of the IAN was not common; therefore, frozen section samples of the neural tissue alone are unlikely to be a representative surrogate of bone margin control.

Cytopathologic techniques and histologic evaluation are complementary techniques that can be used together or individually for the intraoperative evaluation of bone. The advantages of cytopathologic techniques include the ability to collect cells for evaluation from bone margins/specimens that are otherwise awkward to stabilize ex vivo. Collection of cells by the cytobrush technique does not disturb the surface of the bone margin, which will later be evaluated in the formalin-fixed, decalcified state. Cytologic evaluation of cells in a previously irradiated site can be challenging. Histologic evaluation of the medullary bone will remove a portion of the true medullary bone margin when sampled from the specimen, although there is residual bone margin (cortical and remaining medullary bone) remaining for evaluation in the formalin-fixed decalcified state. No false-positive interpretations have been reported for curettings on medullary frozen section analysis, a challenge identified in cytopathologic examination of bone margins (**Fig. 7**).

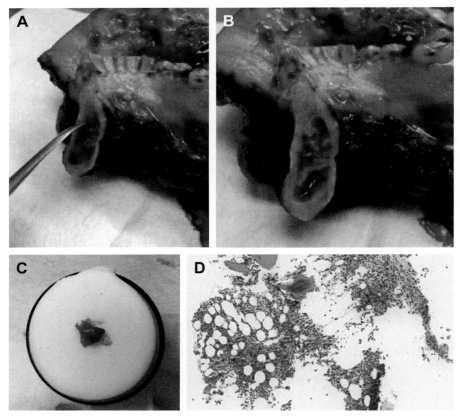

Fig. 7. (*A*) Curettage of the medullary bone margin specimen. (*B*) Appearance of the left mandibular bone margin after medullary sampling for frozen section analysis. (*C*) Medullary bone sample before histologic sectioning during intraoperative consultation with the pathologist. (*D*) Permanent hematoxylin and eosin–stained slide section of the medullary bone margin (H&E stain, original magnification ×70).

SUMMARY

The bone of the jaws and craniofacial skeletal may be the primary site of involvement or secondarily involved by a myriad of benign or malignant neoplasms. Consideration for the nature of the disease, diagnosis, prior therapy, clinical examination, and preoperative imaging are essential data for counseling the patient and planning ablative and, as necessary, reconstructive surgery. Although a complete intraoperative assessment of bone margins continues to represent a technical challenge, the use of cytopathology techniques, histologic evaluation of medullary bone samples, or both when used as complementary techniques, may facilitate intraoperative surgical decision making.

REFERENCES

1. Marchetta FC, Sako K, Murphy JB. The periosteum of the mandible and intraoral carcinoma. Am J Surg 1971;122:711–3.

2. Chen YL, Kuo SW, Fang KH, et al. Prognostic impact of marginal mandibulectomy in the presence of superficial bone invasion and the non-oncologic outcome. Head Neck 2011;33:708–13.
3. Slootweg PJ, Muller H. Mandibular invasion by oral squamous cell carcinoma. J Craniomaxillofac Surg 1989;17:69–74.
4. Ord RA, Sarmadi M, Papadimitrou J. A comparison of segmental and marginal bony resection for oral squamous cell carcinoma involving the mandible. J Oral Maxillofac Surg 1997;55:470–7.
5. Shaw RJ, Brown JS, Woolgar JA, et al. The influence of the pattern of mandibular invasion on recurrence and survival in oral squamous cell carcinoma. Head Neck 2004;26:861–9.
6. OBrien CJ, Adams JR, McNeil EB, et al. Influence of bone invasion and extent of mandibular resection on local control of cancers of the oral cavity and oropharynx. Int J Oral Maxillofac Surg 2003;32:492–7.
7. Genden EM, Rinaldo A, Jacobson A, et al. Management of mandibular invasion: when is a marginal mandibulectomy appropriate? Oral Oncol 2005;41:776–82.

8. Gomez D, Faucher A, Picot V, et al. Outcome of squamous cell carcinoma of the gingiva; a follow-up study of 83 cases. J Craniomaxillofac Surg 2000;28:331–5.

9. Amin MB, Edge SB, Greene FL, et al., AJCC Cancer Staging Manual. 8th Ed. Chicago, Springer 2017.

10. Ebrahimi A, Murali R, Gao K, et al. The prognostic and staging implications of bone invasion in oral squamous cell carcinoma. Cancer 2011;117:4460–7.

11. Okura M, Yanamoto S, Umeda M, et al. Prognostic and staging implications of mandibular canal invasion in lower gingival squamous cell carcinoma. Cancer Med 2016;5:3378–85.

12. Pandey M, Rao LP, Das SR. Predictors of mandibular involvement in cancers of the oromandibular region. J Oral Maxillofac Surg 2009;69:1069–73.

13. Lubek J, El-Hakim M, Salama AR, et al. Gingival carcinoma: retrospective analysis of 72 patients and indications for elective neck dissection. Br J Oral Maxillofac Surg 2011;49:182–5.

14. Overholt SM, Eicher S, Wolf P, et al. Prognostic factors affecting outcome in lower gingival carcinoma. Laryngoscope 1996;106:1335–9.

15. Yamagata K, Ito H, Onizawa K, et al. Prognosis for gingival carcinoma with a delayed diagnosis after dental extraction. J Oral Maxillofac Surg 2013;71:2189–94.

16. Shingaki S, Nomura T, Takada M, et al. Squamous cell carcinomas of the mandibular alveolus: analysis of prognostic factors. Oncology 2002;62:17–24.

17. McGregor AD, MacDonald DG. Routes of entry of squamous cell carcinoma to the mandible. Head Neck Surg 1988;10:294–301.

18. Namin AW, Bruggers SD, Panuganti BA, et al. Efficacy of bone marrow cytologic evaluations in detecting occult cancellous invasion. Laryngoscope 2015;125:E173–9.

19. Sanchis JM, Bagan JV, Murillo J, et al. Mental neuropathy as a manifestation associated with malignant process: its significance in relation to survival. J Oral Maxillofac Surg 2008;66:995–8.

20. Ahuja RB, Soutar DS, Moule B. Comparative study of technetium-99m bone scans and orthopantomography in determining mandible invasion in intraoral squamous cell carcinoma. Head Neck 1990;12:237–43.

21. Acton CHC, Layt C, Gwynne R, et al. Investigative modalities of mandibular invasion by squamous cell carcinoma. Laryngoscope 2000;110:2050–5.

22. Brown JS, Lewis-Jones H. Evidence for imaging the mandible in the management of oral squamous cell carcinoma: a review. Br J Oral Maxillofac Surg 2001;39:411–8.

23. Van Cann EM, Koole R, Oyen WJG, et al. Assessment of mandibular invasion of squamous cell carcinoma by various modes of imaging: constructing a diagnostic algorithm. Int J Oral Maxillofac Surg 2008;37:535–41.

24. Huang SH, Chen CY, Lin WC, et al. A comparative study of fused FDG PET/MRI, PET/CT, MRI and CT imaging for assessing surrounding tissue invasion of advanced buccal squamous cell carcinoma. Clin Nucl Med 2011;36:518–25.

25. Brockenbrough JM, Petruzzelli GJ, Lomasney L. Dentascan as an accurate method of predicting mandibular bone invasion in patients with squamous cell carcinoma of the oral cavity. Arch Otolaryngol Head Neck Surg 2003;129:113–7.

26. Linz C, Muller-Richter UD, Buck AK, et al. Performance of cone beam computed tomography in comparison to conventional imaging techniques for the detection of bone invasion in oral cancer. Int J Oral Maxillofac Surg 2015;44:8–15.

27. Soret M, Bacharach SL, Buvat I. Partial volume effect in PET tumor imaging. J Nucl Med 2007;48:932–45.

28. El-Hafez YGA, Chen CC, Ng SH, et al. Comparison of PET/CT and MRI for the detection of bone marrow invasion in patients with squamous cell carcinoma of the oral cavity. Oral Oncol 2011;47:288–95.

29. Babin E, Desmonts C, Hamon M, et al. PET/CT for assessing mandibular invasion by intraoral squamous cell carcinomas. Clin Otolaryngol 2008;33:47–51.

30. Kim M, Higuchi T, Arisaka Y, et al. Clinical significance of 18F methyltyrosine PET/CT for the detection of bone marrow invasion in patients with oral squamous cell carcinoma: comparison with 18F-FDG PET/CT and MRI. Ann Nucl Med 2013;27:423–30.

31. Van Cann EM, Oyen KJ, Koole R, et al. Bone SPECT reduces the number of unnecessary mandibular resections in patients with squamous cell carcinoma. Oral Oncol 2006;42:409–14.

32. Barttlebort SW, Bahn SL, Ariyan S. Rim mandibulectomy for cancer of the oral cavity. Am J Surg 1987;154:423–8.

33. Guerra MFM, Gias LN, Campo FR, et al. Marginal and segmental mandibulectomy in patients with oral cancer: a statistical analysis of 106 cases. J Oral Maxillofac 2003;61:1289–96.

34. Guerra MFM, Campo FJR, Gias LN, et al. Rim versus sagittal mandibulectomy for the treatment of squamous cell carcinoma: two types of mandibular preservation. Head Neck 2003;25:982–9.

35. Petrovic I, Montero PH, Migliacci JC, et al. Influence of bone invasion on outcomes after marginal mandibulectomy in squamous cell carcinoma of the oral cavity. J Craniomaxillofac Surg 2016;45(2):252–7.

36. Barttelbort SW, Ariyan S. Mandible preservation with oral cavity carcinoma: rim mandibulectomy versus sagittal mandibulectomy. Am J Surg 1993;166:411–5.

37. Brown JS, Griffith JF, Phelps PD, et al. A comparison of different imaging modalities and direct inspection after periosteal stripping in predicting the invasion of

the mandible by oral squamous cell carcinoma. Br J Oral Maxillofac Surg 1994;32:347–59.

38. Wysluch A, Stricker I, Hölzle F, et al. Intraoperative evaluation of bony margins with frozen-section analysis and trephine drill extraction technique: a preliminary study. Head Neck 2010;32(11):1473–8.

39. Weitz J, Pautke C, Wolff KD, et al. Can the inferioralveolar nerve be used as a marker in frozen section for free margin control after segmental mandibulectomy in tumor ablation? Int J Oral Maxillofac Surg 2016;45:1366–71.

40. Mahmood S, Conway DI, Ramesar K. Use of intraoperative cytological assessment of mandibular marrow scrapings to predict resection margin status in patients with squamous cell carcinoma. J Oral Maxillofac Surg 2001;59:1138–41.

41. Nieberer M, Häußler P, Kesting MR, et al. Clinical impact of intraoperative cytological assessment of bone resection margins in patients with head and neck carcinoma. Ann Surg Oncol 2016;23(11): 3579–86.

42. Forrest LA, Schuller DE, Lucas JG, et al. Rapid analysis of mandibular margins. Laryngoscope 1995; 105:475–7.

43. Oxford LE, Ducic Y. Intraoperative evaluation of cortical bony margins with frozen-section analysis. Otolaryngol Head Neck Surg 2006;134: 138–41.

44. Bilodeau EA, Chiosea S. Oral squamous cell carcinoma with mandibular bone invasion: intraoperative evaluation of bone margins by routine frozen section. Head Neck Pathol 2011;5:216–20.

Bone Margin Analysis for Benign Odontogenic Tumors

Eric Ringer, DDS[a], Antonia Kolokythas, DDS, MSc[b],*

KEYWORDS

- Odontogenic tumor • Ameloblastoma • Mandible • Maxilla • Surgical margin

KEY POINTS

- Benign odontogenic tumors can be locally aggressive and may have high recurrence rates if not treated properly.
- Understanding the histology of each subset of tumors can help the surgeon to better understand how recurrence occurs and how best to prevent it.
- When treating benign odontogenic tumors, the surgical margins needed for curative therapy depends on the individual histopathologic diagnosis.
- Although many surgeons opt for conservative therapy, benign odontogenic tumors may need surgical resection.

INTRODUCTION

Benign odontogenic tumors encompass a wide variety of solid and cystic growths that originate from the various components of the odontogenic apparatus. They can be found equally distributed in both genders and in a wide age range, although some do demonstrate prevalence for more particular age groups. Most commonly, these tumors are found incidentally on routine radiographs, because they rarely cause any symptomatology, especially early in their course of development. Occasionally, however, the radiographic investigation is initiated by subjective patient complaints such as tooth loosening or pain, or objective findings such as facial swelling or malocclusion. Despite their benign nature, these tumors tend to behave aggressively in the sense that they can achieve significant sizes even before they become symptomatic, can cause bone and/or root resorption, and some are notorious for their unacceptably high recurrence rates, especially if appropriate treatment is not rendered initially. In addition, these tumors, if neglected or if not treated appropriately, can cause pathologic fractures owing to bone resorption for those found the mandible or extend to adjacent vital structures as the orbit or invade into the skull base, paranasal sinuses, nasal cavity, or infratemporal fossa for those that involve the maxilla.

Treatment of benign odontogenic tumors varies significantly based on the exact histopathologic diagnosis; not all tumors demonstrate the same behavior. Although there is no variation found in the literature regarding the proposed standard treatment of some odontogenic tumors such as the adenomatoid odontogenic tumor, there is significant controversy surrounding the treatment of others, more specifically the odontogenic keratocyst (OKC)/keratocystic odontogenic tumor (KCOT) and the ameloblastoma. Treatment can range from enucleation and curettage to

[a] Department of Oral and Maxillofacial Surgery, University of Rochester-Eastman Institute for Oral Health, 601 Elmwood ave, Box 705, Rochester, NY 14642, USA; [b] Department of Oral and Maxillofacial Surgery, Strong Memorial Hospital, University of Rochester-Eastman Institute for Oral Health, 601 Elmwood Avenue, Box 705, AC-4, Rochester, NY 14642, USA
* Corresponding author.
E-mail address: Antonia_kolokythas@urmc.rochester.edu

Oral Maxillofacial Surg Clin N Am 29 (2017) 293–300
http://dx.doi.org/10.1016/j.coms.2017.03.006
1042-3699/17/

peripheral ostectomy to resection with margins. The traditional teaching is that the tumor that is ameloblastoma or myxoma is treated with resection to the next anatomic layer (periosteum or muscle or fascia) and with a range of linear bony margin. This linear bony margin proposed for resection represents the shortest distance between the pathologic margin and the surgical resection and can range significantly in the literature from 0.5 to 1.5 cm. Interestingly, strict linear margins are often only applied to mandibular resections and not when the tumors involve the maxilla, because vital structures are not commonly sacrificed during maxillary resections for benign pathology. In part, this practice can be attributed to the various histologic subtypes, especially for the ameloblastoma that are believed to behave differently and demonstrate various tumor bone interface characteristics. Equally controversial is the treatment of the OKC/KCOT, specifically regarding the extent of "bony margins" that should be obtained, despite the tremendous body of literature that addresses extensively the histopathologic characteristics and the molecular landscape of the tumor. Finally, unlike in the treatment of malignant pathology, where clear definitions of "free" and "close" margin are established for the various tumors, there is no agreement as to what constitutes a "free" or "close" bony resection margin in benign odontogenic pathology. This article aims to discuss how bony margins are clinically and radiographically evaluated and what is currently known about tumor–bone interface of the most commonly encountered benign odontogenic tumors that guide treatment recommendations specifically regarding the "bony margin" that should be obtained. Although the current literature is depleted of information, we attempt to discuss the various methods that are available to the surgeon for the evaluation of the tumor extent into bone and those that may assist with the preoperative and perioperative assessment of the status of bone margins to ensure adequate tumor resection. The tumors discussed in this article are ameloblastoma, KCOT, odontogenic myxoma, calcifying epithelial odontogenic tumor (CEOT), and adenomatoid odontogenic tumor.

Ameloblastoma

The preoperative assessment of ameloblastoma often begins when first discovered clinically, and fully visualized, most commonly on a panoramic radiograph. Computed tomography (CT) allows for 3-dimensional visualization of the tumor borders and also serves as an indispensable aid in surgical planning specifically for solid tumors.

Traditionally, preoperative imaging has been used to guide the resection plan especially for mandibular tumors since when the tumors involve the maxilla one of the standard maxillectomies (types I–V) is undertaken. Gortzak and colleagues[1] evaluated the borders and spread of ameloblastoma in several patients who underwent resection for large tumors. They found that ameloblastoma invaded via the cancellous bone and had small tumor nests up to 5 mm from the borders of the tumor.

There has been controversy as to the most ideal surgical margin because review of ameloblastoma resections often shows that the tumor extends histologically beyond its radiographic demarcation. Although some have advocated for 3-cm resection margins, and others for enucleation and curettage, the review of most published cases has resulted in the general acceptance of 1.0- to 1.5-cm linear margins for curative treatment.[2–5] In their study of 46 ameloblastomas, Rastogi and colleagues[6] investigated the various histopathologic types of ameloblastomas in an attempt to develop the most effective surgical procedure with curative intent. Using the resection specimens the researchers investigated the bone–tumor interface with serial sections of 0.25 cm. Their study validated that the various histopathologic subtypes of ameloblastoma infiltrate and invade bone differently. They identified that in unicystic ameloblastoma, bony infiltration was seen in 0.25 cm of the bone margin, whereas no tumor was found beyond 0.5 cm. In cases of follicular and plexiform ameloblastoma, tumor was found in up to 0.5 cm of the bone margin, but not beyond 0.75 cm. Finally, in granular ameloblastoma, bone infiltration was found at 0.75 cm of the tumor–bone interface. Based on these findings, they recommended resection of the solid the ameloblastoma variants with 1.0 to 2.0-cm bony margins, but caution against accepting enucleation and curettage as a universal treatment of all cystic tumors. The authors suggest that access to the entirety of the tumor and operator skills best guides the treatment option for the later tumors. One of the limitations of this type of study is that conventional ameloblastoma rarely present in a "pure" form. Instead, it occurs with a mix of histologic appearances. Despite this issue, the concept of treatment based on histopathologic diagnosis is novel. Validation of this study with additional large case series would be very beneficial and perhaps assist in establishing a more defined bony resection margin for each subtype of ameloblastoma that will allow for tumor clearance and prevent unnecessary excision of tumor-free tissue.

Radiographic evaluation of the tumor extent with CT is of paramount importance in assessment and treatment planning. Unfortunately, tumor extension beyond the radiographic margins has been reported to vary significantly with a range between 2 and 8 mm and an average of 4.5 mm. Thus again radiographic margins of 1.0 to 1.5 cm are considered safe and acceptable by many surgeons. This information is widely used for resection planning. The use of intraoperative radiographs of the resected specimen to provide visualization of linear, tumor-free margins has been used to evaluate tumor clearance as well. When the bone resection margins seem to have inadequate linear clearance radiographically, additional bone may be removed or frozen sections may be sent.[7,8] The value of perioperative imaging may be limited for several reasons: tumors located in the anterior mandible and resections that incorporate the parasymphysis region may demonstrate inadequate clearance radiographically simply owing to artifact created by the curvature of the jaw and the manner in which the radiograph was obtained. Maxillary resection specimens are also difficult to assess radiographically, because extensive tumors are often not confined within bone (**Fig. 1**).

In their systematic review of the role of perioperative specimen imaging, de Silva and colleagues[9] identified 1 study that achieved level 4 evidence. The study included 162 tumors over 35 years that were assessed with perioperative specimen imaging after resection.[10] In all studies reviewed, no changes to the resection plan were made based on the findings of the perioperative imaging; neither were any comparisons offered with any other means of margin evaluation. Schaaf and colleagues[11] introduced the utility of perioperative CT in bony specimens of the craniofacial skeleton is discussed. The study included various tumors among those 4 ameloblastomas and overall was found to provide level 4 evidence in supporting the use of perioperative imaging technologies for bone margin evaluation owing to the high-quality images that can be obtained, especially when compared with plain imaging modalities. This could be the most accurate radiographic evaluation of a resected tumor specimen, but may not be readily available and practical for every practitioner. Nevertheless, the surgeon needs to keep in mind the variable tumor extension into the bone and understand that final histopathologic examination of the bone–tumor interface remains the only way to ensure true tumor-free margins.

Intraoperative frozen sections have been used for various reasons to include immediate diagnosis of ameloblastomas, assessment of tumor margins, and more widely used for soft tissue resection margin assessment especially in cases of cortical bone perforation for examination, of the underlying soft tissues.[12] Several investigators, however, have shown the use of frozen sections to assess bony tumor invasion specifically marrow invasion, because ameloblastoma is most often centered within the medullary space. Forrest and colleagues[13] in 1997 showed that frozen section analysis of the bone marrow in malignant disease was negative for tumor and consistent with the final histopathologic examination in 60 margins. Eight bony margins were reported as positive for tumor in frozen sections and again were in agreement with the final histopathologic examination, among those one was an ameloblastoma. The study included 30 cases of mandibular tumors, among them 2 cases of ameloblastoma, the majority were malignant tumors, specifically squamous cell carcinomas. The authors concluded that frozen section analysis of bone margins does have a role in oncologic tumor resection and can be instrumental in intraoperative assessment of margin status and in achieving tumor-free margins. More recently, the literature has shown that incisional biopsy and intraoperative frozen sections have comparable accuracy in the diagnosis of benign intraosseous jaw pathology.[14] Carlson and Marx[8] recommended routine frozen sections for soft tissues, as well as the medullary portion of the resected bone, rather than resecting additional bone without histopathologic examination. It needs to be emphasized that only the marrow can be subjected to frozen sections and not the cortical bone that requires decalcification for

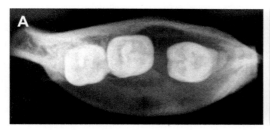 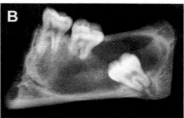

Fig. 1. (*A*, *B*) Radiographic images of resected ameloblastoma specimen.

histopathologic examination. Thus, there are expected limitations of the use of frozen sections for evaluation of bone margins intraoperatively based on the anatomic location of the tumor and the patient as the amount of marrow varies significantly based on location and individual. The comparison of bone marrow frozen sections margins and final histopathologic evaluation specifically for ameloblastoma has yet to be researched with well-designed prospective studies.

If a final pathology report indicates a positive margin postoperatively, a detailed discussion should be held with the patient and consideration to return to the operating room for further resection to excise the tumor completely. Studies have shown that recurrence in "conservative therapy" (ie, enucleation and curettage) ranges from 58% to 93%. In the same studies, recurrence in complete surgical resection ranges from 13% to 15%.[15–17] These data indicate that inadequate surgical margins carry a significant recurrence risk. In patients unwilling or unable to undergo additional surgery, close follow-up with radiographic surveillance and low threshold for biopsy of any suspicious findings could be considered although not the authors' preference. Although the role of radiotherapy for benign odontogenic tumors is yet to be established, there are few studies that have evaluated the use of radiation for positive surgical margins for ameloblastoma and recommend fractionation doses similar to those used for carcinomas.[18]

Odontogenic Keratocyst and Keratocystic Odontogenic Tumor

Similar to most tumors of the maxillofacial skeleton the OKC, synonymously known as KCOT, is often an incidental finding on panoramic radiograph. These radiographs can often be sufficient for the preoperative assessment of the lesion; however, 3-dimensional imaging via CT allows for a more complete understanding of the extent of the lesion, including any bony expansion or perforation through cortical bone. On imaging, an OKC/KCOT will present as a unilocular or multilocular, well-circumscribed radiolucency, occurring most frequently in the posterior mandible.

Reports in the literature regarding recurrence rates of OKC/KCOTs vary, but are generally considered high (25%–60%), mainly owing to specific features associated with the tumor histopathologic and molecular characteristics and the treatment modalities used.[19–21] First, the lining of the OKC/KCOT is extremely thin and friable and often adequate excision cannot be guaranteed, even in small lesions, unless the entire bony cavity hosting the lesion can be visualized directly. Furthermore, lesions may present as multilocular or can be associated with teeth and it is difficult to ensure adequate excision of the cystic lining (**Fig. 2**). Second, daughter cysts often may be present beyond the radiographic and clinical margins of the lesion. Histologic specimens of OKC/KCOT margins may reveal daughter cysts in the surrounding tissues that may contribute to high recurrence rates.[22] Interestingly enough, when enucleation of an odontogenic cystic pathology, such as OKC/KCOT, is performed it is rarely if ever that the pathology report will comment on "margin status" or comment on the integrity of the cystic connective tissue wall. Thus, the presence of cystic components into the surrounding soft tissues cannot be assessed unless resection of these tissues is performed. A third reason for the high recurrence rates may be attributed to the fact that some lesions originate from the oral mucosa and daughter cysts can be found in the overlying mucosa and the cyst. Finally, an important fact that may contribute to the high recurrence rates reported of this pathologic entity is the molecular makeup of the KCOT that explains its aggressive behavior and is the reason for its designation as tumor according to some researchers. Resection for OKC/KCOT, although rarely performed, maybe indicated under specific conditions such as multiple recurrences, extensive soft tissue invasion, and in cases of malignancy, although the latter is an extremely rare event.[23,24] The margins that should be obtained in cases when resection of a KCOT is chosen are not clearly defined in the literature, but it seems that they

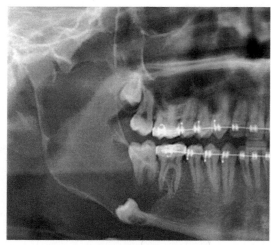

Fig. 2. Portion of panoramic radiograph demonstrating a large radiolucency. Biopsy revealed a keratocystic odontogenic tumor.

would follow those proposed for the other benign odontogenic tumors, such as the ameloblastoma. For the soft tissues that would imply resection to the next anatomic layer, but with regard to the bony margins, the literature lacks studies that critically evaluate what constitutes a safe bone margin.[25–27]

Guthrie and colleagues[14] analyzed the accuracy of frozen section analysis without prior biopsy and examination of biopsy specimens obtained preoperatively in relation to benign intraosseous jaw pathology. They found that the 2 techniques had comparable diagnostic accuracy, but did not examine the use of frozen sections to evaluate adequacy of treatment rendered. In a similar attempt, Aronovich and Kim[12] reviewed the use of intraoperative frozen sections for the diagnosis of benign oral and maxillofacial intrabony lesions as a guide to render treatment in 1 setting. For OKC/KCOTs, the authors found frozen sections to have a sensitivity of 91% and specificity of 98% with regard to obtaining a diagnosis.[12] The study did not evaluate adequacy of excision when final treatment was rendered immediately usually with enucleation and additional removal of bone from the bony cavity directed by either peripheral ostectomy or application of Carnoy's solution or after marsupialization of the lesion. The use of curettage, cryotherapy, or application of Carnoy's solution for the treatment of OKC/KCOT is mainly directed toward ensuring adequate removal of the lesion from the bony cavity and elimination of any lesion residual cystic lining; however, any margin status reported using these techniques is invalidated owing to the lack of specimen that can be submitted or oriented. These approaches aim to remove variable amount of bone, marrow, and cortical bone from the remaining bony cavity to diminish recurrences. The average amount of bone removed with application of Carnoy's solution or cryotherapy is only 1 to 2 mm after various application times. This amount of additional bone removal seems to be universally considered the goal without any studies addressing the exact extension of the lesion into the surrounding bone. The vital structures in the vicinity of the tumor such as the inferior alveolar nerve limit the time that Carnoy's solution should be allowed to be left in the bony cavity. The use of frozen sections examination as the first means of diagnosis may be used to direct the treatment of intrabony pathology and can be critical in reducing surgical time or potentially avoid the need for an incisional biopsy, but in cases of OKC/KCOT it would perhaps be best if this approach could be combined with sampling of the bone margins for frozen section analysis. If enucleation with curettage, cryotherapy, or application of Carnoy's is undertaken as primary treatment of OKC/KCOT it may be beneficial to submit representative margins of the marrow in the remaining bony cavity, similar to what is described in oncologic surgery, in the hopes that frozen sections may assist in determining adequate removal of the lesion. This approach can certainly be technically challenging as it may not yield any information as the "ablative treatment" of the bone may interfere with tissue identification. Despite the vast literature on the behavior of OKC/KCOT, various treatment modalities outcomes, and the biologic nature of this pathologic entity, there is minimal literature specifically evaluating the bone–tumor interface with respect to adequacy of excision.[28,29]

Odontogenic Myxoma

An odontogenic myxoma will typically manifest itself as a unilocular/multilocular, radiolucent lesion with characteristic wispy, bony trabeculation. The preoperative assessment will begin at this time, because the clinician can compare radiographic and clinical findings. A medical-grade or office-based 3-dimensional imagining modality can be used to fully identify the extent of the lesion.

Odontogenic myxoma is characterized by stellate and spindle-shaped cells with long cytoplasmic processes set in a gelatinous, myxoid stroma.[30] Because the lesion is not encapsulated and infiltrates the surrounding tissues, enucleation and curettage is not adequate and will lead to high recurrence rates. A positive surgical margin is present when these soft tissue infiltrations are not completely removed surgically. To prevent recurrence, most have recommended resection with 1.0-cm linear bony margins, confirmed by intraoperative specimen radiography. Similar to other locally invasive odontogenic tumors, it has been recommended to use intraoperative radiographs to confirm appropriate bony margins within a resected specimen.[31–33] The limitations of the use of perioperative plain radiographs to diagnose adequacy of resection margins that are discussed earlier apply to this tumor entity as well. Furthermore, the radiographic delineation of the odontogenic myxoma margins is not as clear as may be the case of the ameloblastoma and the OKC/KCOT (**Fig. 3**). Araki and colleagues[34] offers the most detailed description available of the radiographic appearance of the odontogenic myxoma. The authors state that: "Odontogenic myxoma on radiography tends to display a sharp, thick, straight, trabecular pattern, rather than multilocular septa separated by straight septa forming

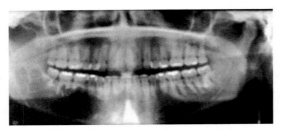

Fig. 3. Panoramic radiograph demonstrating a large multilocular radiolucency of the right mandible. Biopsy revealed odontogenic myxoma.

square, rectangular, or triangular spaces." This detailed radiographic description, if indeed accurate, could be used by the surgeon to plan safe bony resection margins. In addition, the radiographic appearance of the resected specimen could potentially be used to provide more concrete information of the tumor–bone interface that can offer evidence-based guidelines for the resection of odontogenic myxoma.

Because odontogenic myxomas are relatively uncommon tumors, there is limited literature dedicated to the use of frozen sections to assess surgical margin status. Guthrie and colleagues[14] demonstrated that frozen sections can be used to diagnose benign intraosseous jaw pathology with an accuracy comparable with preoperative incisional biopsy. Frozen sections are beneficial in allowing the surgeon to accurately diagnose the lesion and, if appropriate, perform definitive treatment during a single surgery; however, as mentioned, frozen sections were not used to evaluate resection margins.[35] Although not discussed at length in the literature, most case reports indicate that, when a final pathology report reveals a positive surgical margin, further resection should be performed.[36]

Calcifying Epithelial Odontogenic Tumor or Pindborg Tumor

Preoperative evaluation of CEOT begins with the clinical examination. A CEOT is a slow-growing, painless mass. The characteristic radiographic presentation of CEOT is a mixed radiopaque/radiolucent lesion of varying size and opacity, often associated with an impacted tooth. Radiopaque calcifications are usually seen within the radiolucent lesion, described as "driven snow" appearance.[37–39] Although it is often first identified with dental periapical or panoramic radiographs, CT is essential for identification of the extent of the lesion and for surgical planning (**Fig. 4**).

Although there are different histologic variants of CEOT, general histopathologic features usually

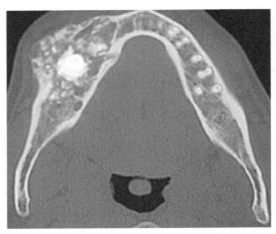

Fig. 4. Axial cut of maxillofacial computed tomography scan demonstrating an extensive radiopaque mass with ill-defined borders extending beyond the buccal cortex. Biopsy revealed a calcifying epithelial odontogenic tumor.

include islands of odontogenic epithelium and amorphous, eosinophilic hyalinized, and acellular regions resembling amyloid. Concentric calcifications are also often present within the amyloid-like areas, termed Leisegang's rings. A positive surgical margin would include these sheets or islands of odontogenic epithelium with bony destruction and calcifications.

Although slow growing, CEOT is locally invasive and destructive. Complete removal is necessary to prevent recurrence.[40] Owing to the small number of reported cases and lack of reliable follow-up for evidence of recurrence, evidence-based recommendations for treatment have not been established. CEOT is generally treated similar to ameloblastoma and odontogenic myxoma by surgical resection with recommended bony linear margins ranging from 0.5 to 1.0 cm.[32,41] Once again, intraoperative radiographs of the resected specimen can be helpful in confirming appropriate margins have been taken. Because it is such an uncommon tumor, with fewer than 200 cases reported, evidence-based literature evaluating frozen sections specifically for CEOT is not available.[12,14]

Management of a positive margin on a final pathology report should encourage serious consideration for further surgical resection. Evaluation of the location and adjacent anatomy should be contemplated, because recurrences can be locally destructive.

Adenomatoid Odontogenic Tumor

The adenomatoid odontogenic tumor is often first identified on routine dental radiographs, and fully visualized via panoramic film or CT. The tumor most commonly presents as a unilocular radiolucency in the anterior maxilla, and is associated with an impacted tooth; CT gives the added benefit of assessing the location and extent of the lesion in a buccal–palatal sense. The surgeon can also palpate the alveolus and evaluate for bony expansion. Appropriate imaging and clinical examination will assist in the choice of access.

Histologically, the adenomatoid odontogenic tumor is composed of spindle or polygonal-shaped cells that form sheets of tissue in a sparse connective tissue stroma. Characteristic ductlike structures are also present throughout the lesion and may contain amorphous eosinic material.[30,42] The tumor itself is contained within a thick, fibrous capsule. A positive margin would indicate that part of this capsule is left behind. There is no distance of margin clearance recommended. The literature supports that, if the fibrous capsule is enucleated completely, the risk of recurrence is negligible.[43] In cases of incomplete removal of the capsule (or a "positive surgical margin") is safely managed postoperatively with long-term radiographic follow-up. As mentioned, however, it is rare that a pathology report will offer information regarding complete removal of the pathologic entity. This is best judged by the surgeon at the time of treatment. There is no information in the current literature regarding the tumor–bone interface that would suggest the need for additional bone removal with curettage or peripheral ostectomy or any other means.

SUMMARY

With the potential exception of the case of ameloblastoma, information relevant to the exact tumor–bone interface and extent of bone invasion by the commonly encountered odontogenic tumors is lacking. These tumors are rare, most likely underreported, and often treated in smaller centers and/or private practice settings. Treatment rendered varies so significantly especially for the smaller sized tumors. Although commonly accepted practices are recommended, scientific evidence is relatively lacking. Prospective multicenter studies from tertiary treatment centers are required to gather adequate data for further investigation of the exact depth of tumor invasion into the adjacent bone and evidence-based guidelines. Some ideas for future studies are offered throughout this article that may help in this direction. Until those studies are available, the proposed linear bone resection margin for odontogenic tumors and the evaluation of its adequacy in tumor eradication will be based on the limited data available.

REFERENCES

1. Gortzak RA, Latief BS, Lekkas C, et al. Growth characteristics of large mandibular ameloblastomas: report of 5 cases with implications for the approach to surgery. Int J Oral Maxillofac Surg 2006;35:691–5.
2. Gold L. Biologic behavior of ameloblastoma. Oral Maxillofac Surg Clin North Am 1991;3:21–71.
3. Nakamura N, Higuchi Y, Mitsuyasu T, et al. Comparison of long-term results between different approaches to ameloblastoma. Oral Surg Oral Med Oral Pathol Oral Radiol Endod 2002;93:13–20.
4. Carlson ER. Ameloblastoma. Symposium on Odontogenic Tumours. AAOMS 82nd Annual Meeting and Scientific Sessions. San Francisco (CA), September 23, 2000.
5. Marx RE, Smith BH, Smith BR, et al. Swelling of the retromolar region and cheek associated with limited opening. J Oral Maxillofac Surg 1993;51:304–9.
6. Rastogi V, Pandilwar PK, Maitra S. Ameloblastoma: an evidence based study. J Maxillofac Oral Surg 2010;9:173–7.
7. Black CC, Addante RR, Mohila CA. Intraosseous ameloblastoma. Oral Surg Oral Med Oral Pathol Oral Radiol Endod 2010;110:585–92.
8. Carlson ER, Marx RE. The ameloblastoma: primary, curative surgical management. J Oral Maxillofac Surg 2006;64:484–94.
9. De Silva I, Rozen WM, Ramakrishnan A, et al. Achieving adequate margins in ameloblastoma resection: the role for intra-operative specimen imaging. Clinical report and systematic review. PLoS One 2012;7:e47897.
10. Keszler A, Paparella ML, Dominguez FV. Desmoplastic and non-desmoplastic ameloblastoma: a comparative clinicopathological analysis. Oral Dis 1996;2:228–31.
11. Schaaf H, Streckbein P, Obert M, et al. High resolution imaging of craniofacial bone specimens by flat-panel volumetric computed tomography. J Craniomaxillofac Surg 2008;36:234–8.
12. Aronovich S, Kim RY. The sensitivity and specificity of frozen-section histopathology in the management of benign oral and maxillofacial lesions. J Oral Maxillofac Surg 2014;72:914–9.
13. Forrest LA, Schuller DE, Karanfilov B, et al. Update on intraoperative analysis of mandibular margins. Am J Otolaryngol 1997;18:396–9.
14. Guthrie D, Peacock ZS, Sadow P, et al. Preoperative incisional and intraoperative frozen section biopsy techniques have comparable accuracy in the diagnosis of benign intraosseous jaw pathology. J Oral Maxillofac Surg 2012;70:2566–72.
15. Sehdev MK, Huvos AG, Strong EW, et al. Proceedings: ameloblastoma of maxilla and mandible. Cancer 1974;33:324–33.

16. Shatkin S, Hoffmeister FS. Ameloblastoma: a rational approach to therapy. Oral Surg Oral Med Oral Pathol 1965;20:421–35.

17. Muller H, Slootweg PJ. The ameloblastoma, the controversial approach to therapy. J Maxillofac Surg 1985;13:79–84.

18. Mendenhall WM, Werning JW, Fernandes R, et al. Ameloblastoma. Am J Clin Oncol 2007;30:645–8.

19. Vedtofte P, Praetorius F. Recurrence of the odontogenic keratocyst in relation to clinical and histological features. A 20-year follow-up study of 72 patients. Int J Oral Surg 1979;8:412–20.

20. Brannon RB. The odontogenic keratocyst. A clinicopathologic study of 312 cases. Part I. Clinical features. Oral Surg Oral Med Oral Pathol 1976; 42:54–72.

21. Pogrel MA. The keratocystic odontogenic tumor. Oral Maxillofac Surg Clin North Am 2013;25:21–30, v.

22. Kolokythas A, Fernandes RP, Pazoki A, et al. Odontogenic keratocyst: to decompress or not to decompress? A comparative study of decompression and enucleation versus resection/peripheral ostectomy. J Oral Maxillofac Surg 2007;65:640–4.

23. Jackson IT, Potparic Z, Fasching M, et al. Penetration of the skull base by dissecting keratocyst. J Craniomaxillofac Surg 1993;21:319–25.

24. Warburton G, Shihabi A, Ord RA. Keratocystic Odontogenic Tumor (KCOT/OKC)-Clinical Guidelines for Resection. J Maxillofac Oral Surg 2015;14: 558–64.

25. Shear M. The aggressive nature of the odontogenic keratocyst: is it a benign cystic neoplasm? Part 3. Immunocytochemistry of cytokeratin and other epithelial cell markers. Oral Oncol 2002;38:407–15.

26. Shear M. The aggressive nature of the odontogenic keratocyst: is it a benign cystic neoplasm? Part 2. Proliferation and genetic studies. Oral Oncol 2002; 38:323–31.

27. Shear M. The aggressive nature of the odontogenic keratocyst: is it a benign cystic neoplasm? Part 1. Clinical and early experimental evidence of aggressive behaviour. Oral Oncol 2002;38:219–26.

28. Johnson NR, Batstone MD, Savage NW. Management and recurrence of keratocystic odontogenic tumor: a systematic review. Oral Surg Oral Med Oral Pathol Oral Radiol 2013;116:e271–6.

29. Blanas N, Freund B, Schwartz M, et al. Systematic review of the treatment and prognosis of the odontogenic keratocyst. Oral Surg Oral Med Oral Pathol Oral Radiol Endod 2000;90:553–8.

30. Reichart PA, Philipsen HP, Sciubba JJ. The new classification of Head and Neck Tumours (WHO)–any changes? Oral Oncol 2006;42:757–8.

31. Simon EN, Merkx MA, Vuhahula E, et al. Odontogenic myxoma: a clinicopathological study of 33 cases. Int J Oral Maxillofac Surg 2004;33:333–7.

32. Miloro M, Ghali GE, Larsen PE, et al. Peterson's principles of oral and maxillofacial surgery. 2nd edition. Hamilton (Canada); London: B C Decker; 2004.

33. Leiser Y, Abu-El-Naaj I, Peled M. Odontogenic myxoma–a case series and review of the surgical management. J Craniomaxillofac Surg 2009;37:206–9.

34. Araki M, Kameoka S, Matsumoto N, et al. Usefulness of cone beam computed tomography for odontogenic myxoma. Dentomaxillofac Radiol 2007;36: 423–7.

35. Subramaniam SS, Heggie AA, Kumar R, et al. Odontogenic myxoma in the paediatric patient: a review of eight cases. Int J Oral Maxillofac Surg 2016;45: 1614–7.

36. Subramaniam S, Nastri A, King J, et al. Endoscopic resection of the pterygoid plates following incomplete transoral resection of an odontogenic myxoma. Br J Oral Maxillofac Surg 2016. [Epub ahead of print].

37. Philipsen HP, Reichart PA. Calcifying epithelial odontogenic tumour: biological profile based on 181 cases from the literature. Oral Oncol 2000;36:17–26.

38. Philipsen HP, Reichart PA. Odontogenic tumors and allied lesions. 1st edition. Hanover Park (IL): Quintessence Publishing Co; 2004.

39. Franklin CD, Pindborg JJ. The calcifying epithelial odontogenic tumor. A review and analysis of 113 cases. Oral Surg Oral Med Oral Pathol 1976;42: 753–65.

40. Kamath G, Abraham R. Recurrent CEOT of the maxilla. Dent Res J (Isfahan) 2012;9:233–6.

41. Maria A, Sharma Y, Malik M. Calcifying epithelial odontogenic tumour: a case report. J Maxillofac Oral Surg 2010;9:302–6.

42. Lee KW. A light and electron microscopic study of the adenomatoid odontogenic tumor. Int J Oral Surg 1974;3:183–93.

43. Philipsen HP, Reichart PA, Zhang KH, et al. Adenomatoid odontogenic tumor: biologic profile based on 499 cases. J Oral Pathol Med 1991;20:149–58.

Bone Margin Analysis for Osteonecrosis and Osteomyelitis of the Jaws

Mohammed Qaisi, DMD, MD[a,b,]*, Lindsay Montague, DMD[c]

KEYWORDS

- Osteonecrosis • MRONJ • Osteomyelitis • ORN • Bone margins • Bisphosphonates • RANKL
- HBO

KEY POINTS

- In advanced osteomyelitis medical and surgical interventions become necessary. Imaging is helpful in preoperative planning.
- In MRONJ, negative margins correlate well with resolution of symptoms. Intraoperative adjuncts, such as fluorescence-guided resection, may become helpful in the future.
- In ORN patients may have persistent disease despite radical resection.
- Margin status on histopathology may not correlate with the clinical outcome.
- High-level evidence data regarding bone margin analysis in osteomyelitis and osteonecrosis of the jaw are lacking. Further studies are needed in this area to help guide treatment and create consensus.

INTRODUCTION

Osteoradionecrosis (ORN), osteomyelitis (OM), and medication-related osteonecrosis of the jaw (MRONJ) are three entities that have a similar appearance clinically, yet are different in their pathophysiology. All three conditions may present with exposed bone within the oral cavity that fails to heal within an 8-week period. The bone can progress to an advanced stage, presenting with suppuration, gross mandibular necrosis, and/or pathologic fractures. Because of their differing pathophysiology, their treatments are also different. The surgical approach to determining margins and subsequent approach to pathologic

bone margin analysis are controversial topics, because of the lack of high-level evidence. This article reviews the available evidence regarding bone margin management and interpretation for each of these entities.

OSTEOMYELITIS

OM is defined as inflammation of the bone and bone marrow caused by an infectious process.[1,2] Some of the etiologies that may result in OM include odontogenic infection, periodontal disease, trauma, inadequate treatment of mandibular fractures, failed mandibular implants or hardware, and hematogenous seeding from bacteremia.[1,3]

[a] Division of Oral & Maxillofacial Surgery, John H. Stroger, Jr. Hospital of Cook County, 1900 West Polk Street, Suite 612, Chicago, IL 60612, USA; [b] Division of Otolaryngology, John H. Stroger, Jr. Hospital of Cook County, 1900 West Polk Street, Suite 612, Chicago, IL 60612, USA; [c] Division Head Oral Pathology, Department of Oral & Maxillofacial Surgery and Pathology, School of Dentistry, University of Mississippi Medical Center, D215, 2500 North State Street, Jackson, MS 39216, USA
* Corresponding author. Division of Oral & Maxillofacial Surgery, John H. Stroger, Jr. Hospital of Cook County, 1900 West Polk Street, Suite 612, Chicago, IL 60612.
E-mail address: moeqaisi@gmail.com

Oral Maxillofacial Surg Clin N Am 29 (2017) 301–313
http://dx.doi.org/10.1016/j.coms.2017.03.007
1042-3699/17/© 2017 Elsevier Inc. All rights reserved.

Patients who have received radiation therapy or medications affecting bone metabolism (discussed later) may have an increased risk for OM.[4] There is a higher predilection for involvement of the mandible likely caused by decreased vascularity when compared with the maxilla. With prevalent use of antibiotics, the incidence of OM has significantly decreased.[1,4] The incidence in the jaws is reported to be around 3 to 4 cases per 100,000 annually.[5,6]

Clinical signs and symptoms associated with OM may include deep boring pain, intraoral or extraoral purulent drainage, intraoral and cutaneous fistula, pathologic fracture, trismus, and neurosensory disturbance.[7]

There is a lack of consensus on a classification system for OM, which may in part be caused by variability in presentation of OM.[8] Several classification systems exist but generally OM is classified as acute or chronic depending on whether the symptoms last over a 1-month period of time.[1] Chronic OM is usually divided into suppurative and nonsuppurative OM.[1,9]

Imaging may be helpful in establishing a diagnosis of OM, determining the extent of disease and subsequent surgical planning.[10] Computed tomography (CT) scan may show a moth-eaten appearance, bony erosion, sequestration, gross bony destruction, or any combination of these features. MRI may detect earlier stages of OM showing hypointensity of the marrow on T1-weighted images, and hyperintensity on T2 postcontrast images, signifying medullary inflammation. These changes appear on MRI before the occurrence of cortical osseous changes, making the MRI more sensitive and specific in the acute phase.[11–13] The most common nuclear medicine imaging techniques involves bone scintigraphy using a radiopharmaceutical tracer diphosphonates coupled to the radionuclide technetium-99m (^{99m}Tc). The tracer selectively accumulates on bone mineral matrix in areas of high metabolic/osteoblastic activity. This test is sensitive but not specific and can be positive in cases of trauma, tumors, and aseptic conditions. Autologous tagged white blood cell (leukoctyes) scitingraphy can help to localize the source as leukocytes accumulate by migration toward the bone infection. Another drawback to nuclear testing includes the time required (hours) and the poor image quality because of the spatial resolution of the gamma camera with the inability to detect bone sequestra less than 8 mm. Combined with other imaging modalities, such as single-photon emission CT or PET-CT, imaging can further improve the diagnostic yield and localize the infection.[14,15]

There is currently no consistent protocol or accepted guideline in the literature for the treatment of OM.[8] Most therapeutic recommendations are based of the findings of single reports or textbooks. Cases limited in extent, and/or cases of acute OM, may be managed with antibiotics with or without surgery. In chronic OM, surgical intervention is required in combination with antibiotics. The extent and type of surgical treatment depends on presentation and may include conservative debridement and/or sequestrectomy. Decortication and saucerization of the involved area of the mandible has also been reported to be successful in certain cases of OM.[16] Segmental resection is reserved for advanced cases of OM that fail medical therapy and demonstrate gross necrosis of the mandible, suppuration, draining cutaneous fistula, intractable pain, and/or pathologic fracture (**Fig. 1**).[1,4]

When segmental resection is deemed necessary for treatment, general consensus recommendation suggests a 1-cm bone margin beyond the identifiable boundary of the radiographic process when feasible. Additional bone should be resected if bleeding bone (a clinical surrogate for viability) is not observed.[4,17] Although evidence-based research regarding the placement of the most appropriate margin for resection of mandibular OM is lacking, there seems to be good correlation between cross-sectional radiographic studies and pathologic bony margins.[10] This correlation between preoperative imaging and accurate final pathologic bone margin status allows for ease in preoperative ablative and reconstructive planning. Microvascular free flap reconstruction is also helpful because it allows the surgeon the ability to attain generous resection margins with healthy viable bone (see **Fig. 1**).

Antibiotics are required in addition to surgery in the management of OM.[4] Kim and Jang[16] showed 95% control rates for OM when using surgery and 8 weeks of antibiotic therapy, compared with control rates of 60% in the surgery alone arm. Again, there is a lack of consensus with regards to the type and route of antibiotics to be used and the length of therapy.[8] These cases are best treated in a multidisciplinary fashion with infectious disease specialists, with individualized treatment being based on tissue cultures and clinical response.[2,4] The most commonly cultured microbes include normal oral flora, staphylococcus, and bacteroides.[16,18] Because it is important to select an appropriate antibiotic, one must remember that deep tissue cultures or marrow cultures from the specimen should be attained before the main specimen being immersed in formalin and sent to pathology.

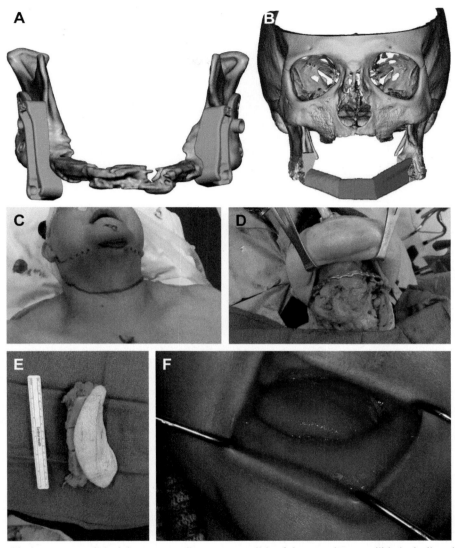

Fig. 1. Mandibular osteomyelitis. (*A*) Long-standing osteomyelitis of the anterior mandible including the planned osteotomies. (*B*) Planned reconstruction with fibula free flap. (*C*) Submental chronic draining fistula and planned fistulectomy. (*D*) After mandibular resection and placement of reconstruction bar. (*E*) Fibula free flap before inset and anastomosis. (*F*) Three months postoperative. Intraoral view showing mucosalization of skin paddle.

Microscopically, biopsy and resection specimens of OM are composed of necrotic bone with empty osteocyte lacunae, peripheral resorption, and acute or chronic inflammatory infiltrates (**Fig. 2**A).[19] The bone sequestrum may demonstrate microorganisms on the surface (**Fig. 2**B) or within the marrow spaces, often morphologically suggestive of an *Actinomyces* species.[4] As the infection progresses into the chronic stages, reactive viable bone formation with irregular basophilic reversal lines (**Fig. 3**) may be observed.[4,20] The resection margins may exhibit normal or sclerotic viable bone, nonviable bone, or a mixture of new and necrotic bone.

The ability to accurately report the margin status in gnathic OM depends on the treatment and the resultant surgical pathology specimen, and good communication between the surgeon and the pathologist. For cases treated with debridement or curettage, the specimen is received by the laboratory as multiple fragments of unoriented bone, precluding accurate margin evaluation. In cases treated with marginal or segmental resection, intact specimens or those with separately submitted margins (eg, anterior, posterior) allow for histopathologic margin evaluation. When examining the bone margins, it may be helpful to subsequent

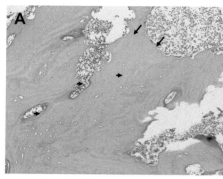
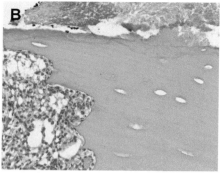

Fig. 2. Suppurative osteomyelitis. (*A*) Nonviable bone with empty lacunae (*arrowheads*), resorption by osteoclasts (*arrows*), and inflammation within the marrow space (hematoxylin-eosin [H&E], original magnification ×100). (*B*) Higher magnification from another area in same specimen as *A* showing neutrophils and bacterial colonization of the surface of the necrotic bone (H&E, original magnification ×400).

treating physicians for the pathologist to report evidence of overtly necrotic bone and/or acute inflammation or abscess at the bone margin, versus finding scant chronic inflammation and/or viable bone devoid of inflammation.

In many institutions, categoric classification of bone margin status (positive or negative) or even descriptive findings (previous paragraph) are not routinely reported by pathologists in cases of resected gnathic OM, which limits the study of this disease, and correlation of pathologic and surgical variables contributing to recurrence. This may be caused by a multitude of reasons including specimen fragmentation, an institutional or pathologist bias where margin interpretation is not viewed as necessary in a benign and/or infectious process, lack of communication between surgeon and pathologist, or the submission of unoriented specimens may signal that margin analysis is not required. Therefore it is imperative for surgeons to indicate that bony margin analysis is required and to orient specimens even if orientation of the specimen seems obvious to the surgeon.

Although persistence of disease may be related to residual necrotic bone, there are no specific articles in the literature regarding the importance of microscopically viable bone margins in OM of the mandible and maxilla. In the diabetic foot, studies have shown that patients with positive resection margins via histopathology or bone culture had poor outcomes, often requiring further surgery.[21–23] The applicability of these findings to cases of jaw OM may be limited because of differences in anatomy, vascularity, type of bacteria (when present), patient comorbidities, or other factors unique to the maxilla and mandible. Further studies are needed to determine the clinical significance of microscopically negative bone margin status in gnathic OM.

MEDICATION-RELATED OSTEONECROSIS

Antiresorptive medications including bisphosphonates and receptor activator of nuclear factor kappa-B ligand (RANKL) inhibitors have been used in the treatment of distant bony metastasis, as in the cases of breast and prostate cancer,

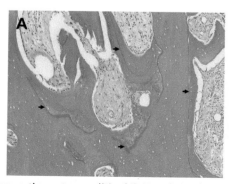
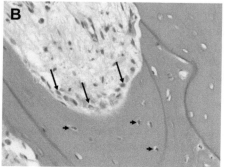

Fig. 3. Suppurative osteomyelitis. (*A*) New bone being laid down on top of nonviable bone with prominent reversal lines (*arrowheads*) (H&E, original magnification ×100). (*B*) Higher magnification of *A* showing osteoblastic rimming (*arrows*) and viable osteocytes (*arrowheads*) (H&E, original magnification ×400).

and in the prevention of osteoporosis.[24,25] Both drug classes are available in oral and parenteral formulations depending on the indication. Bisphosphonates have been used for more than 40 years, whereas RANKL inhibitors have only been approved by the Food and Drug Administration since 2010.[25,26] Although these drugs fulfill their intended purpose of effectively reducing skeletal-related events in these patients, an important side effect in the maxillofacial region is development of MRONJ. MRONJ is defined as exposure of bone for a period greater than 8 weeks in a patient on or with a history of antiresorptive medication use, and no prior history of radiation therapy.[27] An overview of all the antiresorptive and antiangiogenic agents that result in MRONJ is beyond the scope of this text and the reader is encouraged to refer to the position paper provided by the American Association of Oral and Maxillofacial Surgery.[24]

Although the mechanism of action of these medications has not been fully elucidated, the negative impact on osteoclast function and thus bone turnover is widely accepted.[28–30] Bisphosphonates covalently bind to bone accounting for its very slow elimination from the body, often persisting in bone for several years after the cessation of the drug. Conversely, RANKL inhibitors have a much shorter half-life of 25 to 30 days with its effects dissipating within 6 months of cessation of treatment.[31] Risk factors for development of MRONJ include the duration of therapy, cumulative dose, and the type of antiresorptive medication used.[32,33] The most commonly identified trigger for MRONJ is invasive dental surgery, such as dental extractions. At present, MRONJ is classified based on severity, ranging from stage 0 to stage 3. Stage 3 involves the entire thickness of the mandible, and may present with signs to include neck fistula, purulence expression, and or pathologic fracture.[24,27]

Treatment depends on the stage and progression of the disease but remains controversial. Although many authors advocate for conservative intervention and localized measures for patients with stage 1 and 2 disease,[24,34–37] others advocate resection with clear margins.[38,39] Carlson and Basile advocate for surgical resection, either marginal or segmental resection as dictated by the ability to generate clear margins, irrespective of the stage. The authors report that this approach has yielded good results with resolution of symptoms.[37]

Segmental mandibular resection is typically reserved for patients with advanced stage 3 disease, and has been shown to result in resolution of symptoms.[24,38] Resection should be planned for 1 cm beyond the involved bone based on

preoperative CT and MRI imaging.[40] Resection to bleeding bone is prerequisite to predict favorable bone and soft tissue healing.[39] Pautke and colleagues[41] reported their experience with intraoperative fluorescence-guided resection to help assess adequate surgical margins. Tetracycline is administered for 10 days before the procedure and a fluorescence lamp is used intraoperatively. Because tetracycline is absorbed only by viable bone, bone removal is carried out until all the dark necrotic bone is removed, leaving behind a homogenous green fluorescent viable bone. This showed 85% success rate in a prospective descriptive pilot study. Autofluorescence, using the lamp without the preoperative tetracycline, has also been reported to be helpful in guiding surgical decision making.[42]

Another factor that should be taken into consideration is the quality of the overlying gingival tissue and the negative effect bisphosphonates have on oral mucosal healing.[24] For that reason it may be strategic to place osteotomies in areas with robust vascularized soft tissue covering, such as the pterygomasseteric sling, and to avoid osteotomies within 1 cm of a tooth.[39] If a fibula free flap is used to reconstruct a continuity defect, either a skin paddle or an adequate length of muscle should also be harvested to reline the oral cavity with adequate soft tissue coverage in a tension-free fashion to minimize bone exposure postreconstruction. Despite the diffuse uptake of antiresorptive medications in the body, resection and fibula free flap reconstruction seems successful in eradicating MRONJ in more than 90% of cases, provided negative margins are obtained.[43] The fibula is rarely the site of metastatic bone disease or multiple myeloma, when compared with the ileum or scapula, and therefore could be considered a first-line flap for reconstruction in MRONJ cases.[43] PET imaging or bone scan should be obtained to assess donor site viability and rule out the transfer of a metastatic deposit to the newly reconstructed jaws. Furthermore, because of the diffuse uptake antiresorptive medications, subtotal mandibulectomy is sometimes needed to clear the involved bone as demonstrated in a series of seven patients by Nocini and colleagues[38,43] One must carefully examine the mandible clinically and radiographically, to ensure that the disease is localized before embarking on a unilateral resection, because the possibility of multifocal disease secondary to the systemic effect of the drug may explain why subtotal mandibulectomy is prevalent in some series (**Figs. 4** and **5**).[43]

Although there is no evidence to recommend a temporary cessation of bisphosphonate medication (drug holiday) before undergoing surgical

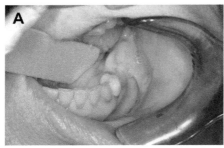
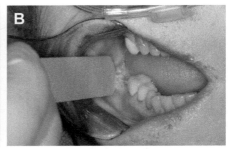

Fig. 4. MRONJ with multifocal exposure. (*A*) Patient with history of denosumab (Prolia) use for osteoporosis. Notice multifocal nature of disease with left posterior mandible exposure and small exposure in the anterior mandible. (*B*) There is small exposure and minimal suppuration in the right posterior mandible.

resection of MRONJ-related diseased tissue, many prescribing physicians endorse this for their patients.[36,39,43] Bisphosphonates are incorporated into the matrix of the skeleton for years, but on balance, RANKL inhibitors are almost completely eliminated from the body after a period 6 months. Based on the latter, one may hypothesize that a drug holiday maybe helpful in these situations.[31] Further studies need to validate this hypothesis.

The histopathology of MRONJ shows overlap with OM and ORN. Similar to OM and ORN, portions of the affected bone in MRONJ are devoid of osteocytes and osteoblasts and lack normal bone marrow cells.[18,44] MRONJ specimens tend to lack the inflammatory infiltrates seen in OM or the marrow fibrosis seen in ORN (**Fig. 6**A), unless superinfected or pathologic fracture has occurred.[20] The periphery of the bone in areas of active MRONJ is often irregular with evidence of resorption and detached or absent osteoclasts.[27,43,45] Exposed bone and sequestrum exhibit bacterial colonization of the surface, most often morphologically consistent with an *Actinomyces* species, whereas the overlying mucosa may demonstrate pseudoepitheliomatous hyperplasia and inflammation (**Fig. 6**B).[46] In regions of

viable bone, hyperemia and inflammatory infiltrates may be noted in the marrow spaces (**Fig. 7**A) and new bone formation or periosteal reaction may be observed.[45] The bone may also exhibit a pagetoid pattern with prominent basophilic reversal lines and enlarged or irregular osteoclasts in viable areas (**Fig. 7**B).[19] Overall, MRONJ specimens tend to exhibit a mixed pattern of necrosis with areas of lamellar bone containing viable osteocytes adjacent to areas with empty lacunae.[44]

In a multicenter retrospective review, Carlson and colleagues[47] identified microscopic evidence of malignancy in 5.3% of biopsies and resection specimens of patients clinically diagnosed with MRONJ. Therefore, bony specimens require thorough sampling to exclude deposits of malignancy contributing to the underlying bone destruction, which may be radiographically undetectable in the background of osteonecrosis.[38–40] Where surgical margin status can be determined, the pathologist could consider reporting several data points when observed at the bony surgical margins including the presence or absence of organisms, nature of the inflammatory response (acute or chronic), and if malignancy is detected within the specimen, then an assessment of adequacy in

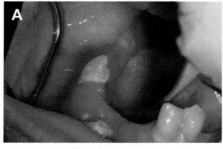
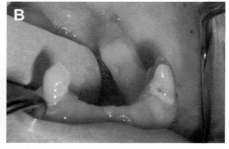

Fig. 5. MRONJ with multifocal bone exposure. (*A*) Patient with previous history of bisphosphonate use for breast cancer. Notice multifocality of involvement with exposed bone in the anterior mandible and pinpoint exposure along the right myelohyoid ridge. (*B*) Showing exposure along left myelohyoid ridge.

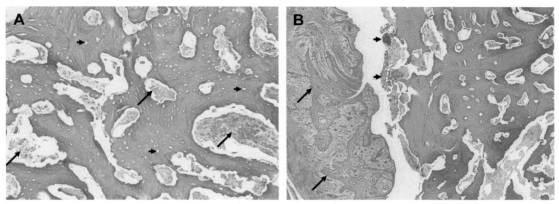

Fig. 6. Medication-related osteonecrosis. (*A*) Necrotic bone with empty lacunae (*arrowheads*), peripheral resorption, and marrow spaces containing bacterial colonies (*arrows*), but lacking inflammation or fibrosis (H&E, original magnification ×100). (*B*) Area of bone exposed to oral cavity showing epithelial hyperplasia (*arrows*) adjacent to necrotic bone with *Actinomyces* bacterial colonization (*arrowheads*) (H&E, original magnification ×100).

relation to the specimen margin. The histopathologic findings in resection specimens seem to correlate well with CT and MRI findings, allowing for removal of affected bone with uninvolved margins, despite the diffuse nature of the disease, in most cases.[44]

Specimens obtained by some forms of surgical intervention for MRONJ, such as debridement and sequestrectomy, are not amenable to accurate margin reporting because these specimens are received fragmented, unoriented, and portions of the specimen may be diverted for culture and/or other testing. In cases where a surgical resection has been performed with the expectation that a pathologic evaluation of margin status will be provided, there is no consensus on which parameters are prognostically relevant for reporting. In comparison with OM and ORN, which may develop in bones other than the jaws, MRONJ tends to favor the gnathic bones, which limits extrapolation of

research data from other anatomic sites. This lack of data, and possible multifocality of disease, makes it even more challenging to correlate margin status and clinical course. Studies specifically examining the relationship of margins and clinical outcome have found that patients with "normal bone" present at the resection margins demonstrated good long-term disease control and those with margins exhibiting "osteomyelitis" developed recurrent MRONJ within 3 to 6 months of follow-up.[38,43]

OSTEORADIONECROSIS

ORN is clinically defined by exposed bone for more than 2 months in a previously radiated area without prior history of antiresorptive medication use.[48–51] ORN is a side effect of radiation therapy and is more likely to occur when the dose of radiation to the mandible exceeds 60 Gy.[52] The

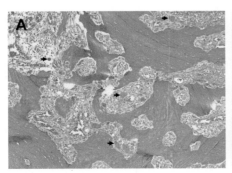
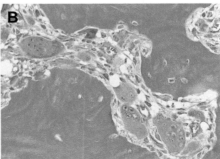

Fig. 7. Medication-related osteonecrosis. (*A*) Margin of resection specimen showing areas of viable bone with inflamed, vascular marrow spaces and numerous osteoclasts (*arrowheads*) (H&E, original magnification ×100). (*B*) Higher magnification of *A* showing enlarged osteoclasts and osteocytes within lacunae (H&E, original magnification ×400).

incidence of ORN has decreased over the years from an estimated 15% in the 1970s to 0% to 5% in the 2000s. Some of this might be attributed to advances in radiation therapy and the improved dose distribution of intensity-modulated radiation therapy.[53–56]

Clinical presentation may vary based on stage, ranging from an asymptomatic area of exposed bone increasing in severity to include gross bone necrosis involving the full thickness and height of the mandible with pathologic fracture (**Fig. 8**). Other associated clinical signs and symptoms may include dysesthesia, pain, malodor, swelling, ulcerations, suppuration, and trismus.[48,57] Radiographically ORN can show findings that are indistinguishable from the two entities described previously. These include areas of osteolysis and resorption extending to the inferior mandibular border, bone sequestration, increased bone opacification, and mottling.[1]

ORN is classified as stage 1 through 3 based on severity and extent of involvement. The two most commonly used staging systems are the ones described by Marx[51] and Notani and colleagues[58] (**Table 1**). The exact pathophysiology of ORN remains controversial.[48] Marx's 3-H theory proposes direct damage by ionizing radiation leading to hypoxia, hypocellularity, and hypovascularity.[51] This theory led to the adoption of hyperbaric oxygen (HBO) in the treatment algorithm of ORN. The protocol usually involves 20 to 30 dives at 2.4 atmospheric pressure before a surgical intervention or dental extraction and an additional 10 dives afterward.[59,60] Although a few early studies examining the role of HBO in the treatment of ORN showed promise, more recent data have been less supportive, and there remains a paucity of evidence in support of HBO in the treatment of ORN.[61,62] A recent multicenter randomized

double-blinded clinical trial examining the use of HBO in the treatment of ORN was discontinued before the conclusion of the study because of worse outcomes in the HBO group compared with the placebo group.[60] Although criticized for design flaws, this study has led to the questioning of the 3-H theory and the role HBO therapy in ORN.[48,57,63] Others authors reported higher perioperative complications when performing segmental resection with microvascular reconstruction in patients previously treated with HBO when compared with HBO-naive patients.[64]

A competing theory for the pathogenesis of ORN by Delanian and colleagues[65] suggests radiation-induced fibrosis as the mechanism of injury. Cells in the bone are damaged as a result of acute inflammation, free radicals, and the chronic activation and dysregulation of fibroblasts leading to matrix densification and tissue necrosis.[64] Based on this, pentoxifylline and tocopherol in synergy have been shown to be effective in the treatment of ORN through their antioxidant and antifibrotic effects.[65] A second phase II trial confirmed these results showing the combination of pentoxifylline, tocopherol, and clodronate to be effective in the treatment of refractory ORN, inducing mucosal and bone healing with significant symptom improvement.[66] A histopathologic study by Marx and Tursun[20] in 2012 showed marrow fibrosis in ORN specimens, which could be interpreted to be in line with this theory.

Early stage disease and asymptomatic patients can be managed conservatively with oral care, antibiotics if necessary, and the use of pentoxifylline and tocopherol.[65] Some advocate for the use of these medications prophylactically before and after dental extractions, in a fashion similar to the way HBO was traditionally used.[57] Debridement, curettage, and sequestrectomy may be used

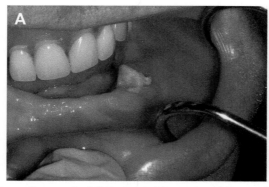
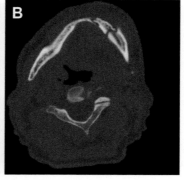

Fig. 8. Osteoradionecrosis. (*A*) Patient with previous history of irradiation to the oral cavity. Notice the bony exposure intraorally in the left mandible. (*B*) Axial cut CT scan showing radiographic changes in the left mandible with presence of a pathologic fracture.

Table 1
Notani classification system for ORN

Notani Class	Features
Class I	ORN confined to alveolar bone
Class II	ORN of alveolar bone and/or mandible *above* the level of the inferior alveolar canal
Class III	ORN involving the mandible *below* the level of the inferior alveolar canal, presence of cutaneous fistula, or pathologic fracture

Adapted from Notani K, Yamazaki Y, Kitada H, et al. Management of mandibular osteoradionecrosis corresponding to the severity of osteoradionecrosis and the method of radiotherapy. Head Neck 2003;25:181–6; with permission.

when there is clinical evidence of a sequestrum, or if the patient is symptomatic.[67] These specimens are submitted to pathology for microscopic evaluation, although portions may be considered for culture in the correct clinical context. There is no expectation of a formal pathologic margin status evaluation.

Advanced ORN as identified by marked necrosis, pathologic fracture, or orocutaneous fistulas is best treated with segmental resection and microvascular reconstruction.[67–70] Microvascular free tissue transfer not only allows for reconstruction of the bony defect, but also provides for healthy soft tissue to help with tension-free closure of heavily irradiated, fibrotic inelastic skin that would be otherwise difficult to close primarily. Resection is usually planned with a 1-cm margin beyond the radiographic changes or until bleeding and healthy-appearing bone is reached.

As with the case of MRONJ and OM, there is minimal evidence to guide the surgical placement of bone margins. One recent report found that approximately 25% of patients with mandibular ORN developed recurrent disease despite extensive mandibular resection.[71] A subsequent follow-up study by the same authors attempted to correlate histologic findings of surgical bone margins with progression of ORN. In this study, Zaghi and colleagues[72] evaluated 34 patients treated with radical resection of the mandible and found no correlation between residual necrotic bone margins and persistent disease. Of the 26 cases with histologically negative margins for necrosis, eight developed progression of ORN. The authors reported that of the eight patients who were identified to have positive bone necrosis at the margins on initial histologic evaluation, none showed evidence of persistent disease at follow-up visits. Additional studies are needed to identify clinical parameters that impact placement of surgical margins, in addition to identification of histologic variables within the specimen and at the margin that better correlate with clinical outcome.

Maurer and Meyer[73] reported a case in which ORN resection was guided by the partial pressure of oxygen (Po_2) within the bone measured using a fine-needle Eppendorf probe, measured via bur holes drilled into the mandible. In prior work, the investigators established a partial pressure value of greater than 71.7 mm Hg as a surrogate for healthy bone, whereas values less than 32.3 were consistent with ORN. Although novel, no additional studies examining this technique have been published since the initial case report in 2006. Similar to MRONJ, tetracycline bone fluorescence was found to be helpful as an adjunct in guiding intraoperative resection margins in

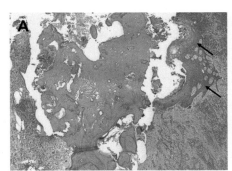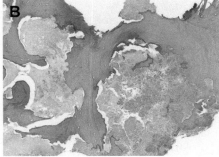

Fig. 9. Osteoradionecrosis. (*A*) Surface of necrotic bone exposed to oral cavity with pseudoepitheliomatous hyperplasia (*arrows*), inflammation, and fibrosis of the mucosa (H&E, original magnification ×40). (*B*) Another area from same specimen as *A* showing peripheral resorption of the necrotic bone by aggregates of *Actinomyces* bacteria (H&E, original magnification ×100).

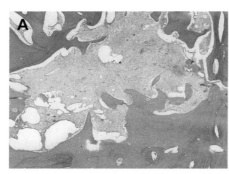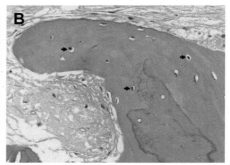

Fig. 10. Osteoradionecrosis. (*A*) Mandibular resection margin showing fibrous replacement of the marrow in an area of viable bone (H&E, original magnification ×40). (*B*) Higher magnification of *A* demonstrating osteocytes within lacunae (*arrowheads*) (H&E, original magnification ×400).

ORN according to a single case report.[74] Other reports have shown the use of near infrared fluorescence for the evaluation of bony margins. Indocyanine green dye is injected intravenously and the perfusion to bony margins is assessed using a portable infrared imager.[75] Further studies are needed to validate all of these adjuncts.

On histologic evaluation, specimens of ORN demonstrate death of osteocytes with empty lacunae and lack of osteoblastic rimming, similar to OM and MRONJ.[18,51] The overlying mucosa may demonstrate pseudoepitheliomatous hyperplasia in the areas where the bone is exposed to the oral cavity (**Fig. 9**A), and fibrosis of the connective tissue with decreased cellularity and vascularity.[45,51,76] In ORN and MRONJ, the *Actinomyces* microorganisms are usually seen on the surface of the bone exposed to the oral cavity (**Fig. 9**B), rather than throughout the bone, as is the case with suppurative OM.[18,49] The pattern of bone necrosis in ORN is appreciated in resection specimens or large biopsies. In ORN, the pattern is reported as uniform in appearance with large areas of necrosis and empty lacunae, whereas in MRONJ the necrosis is often patchy with alternating areas of viable and nonviable bone.[46,76] These features may be obscured by prior instrumentation, superinfection, and/or pathologic fracture. ORN tends to demonstrate more significant fibrosis of the marrow (**Fig. 10**A) with an absence of normal marrow elements and lack of functioning blood vessels or inflammatory cells, when compared with suppurative OM or MRONJ.[20] At the resection margins, the bone may appear viable with visible osteocytes within lacunae (**Fig. 10**B) and blood vessels within haversian canals, or necrotic with empty lacunae and canals.[72]

Most patients with ORN have a prior history of malignancy; therefore, careful sampling of the specimen for recurrent, metastatic or posttreatment

malignancy is imperative. In a retrospective review by Marwan and colleagues,[77] 2.48% of patients had microscopic evidence of malignancy in the resection specimen of cases presumed to be ORN.

When a surgical resection has been performed with the expectation that a pathologic evaluation of margin status will be provided, traditional histologic parameters might include presence or absence of necrosis, inflammation, nature of the inflammatory response (acute or chronic), and the presence or absence of malignancy at the margin. The lack of concordance between absence of necrosis and progression of disease identified by Zaghi and colleagues[72] suggests additional clinical and histologic prognostic parameters should be explored.

SUMMARY

Bone margin analysis in cases of OM, ORN, and MRONJ is a controversial topic. As discussed in this article, there is a paucity of evidence to guide therapy and interpretation of bone margins. Using imaging in planning surgery seems to be helpful, because often the radiographic changes are more extensive than what is seen clinically. Intraoperative adjuncts, such as tetracycline fluorescence, show some promise in margin assessment for surgical management of MRONJ, although this needs to be evaluated further. Other adjuncts including infrared fluorescence, autofluorescence, and the use of bone Po_2 measurements have been reported in case reports only, and need to be investigated further. Obtaining clear margins seems to correlate with better outcomes in OM and MRONJ, but this was not demonstrated in ORN. Nonetheless, one should attempt to obtain clear margins whenever feasible. Pathologists are encouraged to evaluate and report on bony margins in these entities as they would for malignant disease. This would allow for better understanding of the clinical outcomes in these patients, and allows for the possibility of future studies. Likewise, it is important that surgeons communicate with their pathology colleagues, indicate that bone margin analysis is required, and orient surgical specimens even when orientation of the specimen seems obvious.

REFERENCES

1. Kushner G, Alpert B. Osteomyelitis and osteoradionecrosis. In: Miloro M, Ghali G, Larsen P, et al, editors. Peterson's principles of oral & maxillofacial surgery, vol. 1, 2nd edition. London: BC Decker Inc; 2004. p. 313–23.

2. Bamberger DM. Osteomyelitis. A commonsense approach to antibiotic and surgical treatment. Postgrad Med 1993;94:177–82, 184.

3. Bevin CR, Inwards CY, Keller EE. Surgical management of primary chronic osteomyelitis: a long-term retrospective analysis. J Oral Maxillofac Surg 2008; 66:2073–85.

4. Krakowiak PA. Alveolar osteitis and osteomyelitis of the jaws. Oral Maxillofacial Surg Clin N Am 2011; 23:401–13.

5. Bronkhorst MA, van Damme PA. Osteomyelitis of the jaws. Ned Tijdschr Tandheelkd 2006;113:222–5 [in Dutch].

6. Koorbusch GF, Fotos P, Goll KT. Retrospective assessment of osteomyelitis. Etiology, demographics, risk factors, and management in 35 cases. Oral Surg Oral Med Oral Pathol 1992;74:149–54.

7. Hudson JW. Osteomyelitis of the jaws: a 50-year perspective. J Oral Maxillofac Surg 1993;51:1294–301.

8. Walter G, Kemmerer M, Kappler C, et al. Treatment algorithms for chronic osteomyelitis. Dtsch Arztebl Int 2012;109:257–64.

9. Lew DP, Waldvogel FA. Osteomyelitis. N Engl J Med 1997;336:999–1007.

10. Tanaka R, Hayashi T. Computed tomography findings of chronic osteomyelitis involving the mandible: correlation to histopathological findings. Dentomaxillofac Radiol 2008;37:94–103.

11. Schuknecht BF, Carls FR, Valavanis A, et al. Mandibular osteomyelitis: evaluation and staging in 18 patients, using magnetic resonance imaging, computed tomography and conventional radiographs. J Craniomaxillofac Surg 1997;25:24–33.

12. Love C, Patel M, Lonner BS, et al. Diagnosing spinal osteomyelitis: a comparison of bone and Ga-67 scintigraphy and magnetic resonance imaging. Clin Nucl Med 2000;25:963–77.

13. Schuknechi B. Diagnostic Imaging - conventional radiology, computed tomography, and magnetic resonance imaging. In: Baltensperger M, Eyrich G, editors. Osteomyelitis of jaws. Berlin: Springer; 2009. p. 57–94.

14. Love C, Palestro CJ. Nuclear medicine imaging of bone infections. Clin Radiol 2016;71:632–46.

15. Pineda C, Espinosa R, Pena A. Radiographic imaging in osteomyelitis: the role of plain radiography, computed tomography, ultrasonography, magnetic resonance imaging, and scintigraphy. Semin Plast Surg 2009;23:80–9.

16. Kim SG, Jang HS. Treatment of chronic osteomyelitis in Korea. Oral Surg Oral Med Oral Pathol Oral Radiol Endod 2001;92:394–8.

17. Topazian R. Osteomyelitis of jaws. In: Topazian R, Goldberg M, Hupp J, editors. Oral & maxillofacial infections. 4th edition. Philadelphia: Saunders; 2002. p. 214–42.

18. Gentry LO. Osteomyelitis: options for diagnosis and management. J Antimicrob Chemother 1988; 21(Suppl C):115–31.

19. Chi A. Pulpal and periapical disease. In: Neville B, Damm D, Allen C, et al, editors. Oral & maxillofacial pathology. 4th edition. St Louis (MO): Elsevier; 2016. p. 128–39.

20. Marx RE, Tursun R. Suppurative osteomyelitis, bisphosphonate induced osteonecrosis, osteoradionecrosis: a blinded histopathologic comparison and its implications for the mechanism of each disease. Int J Oral Maxillofac Surg 2012;41:283–9.

21. Kowalski TJ, Matsuda M, Sorenson MD, et al. The effect of residual osteomyelitis at the resection margin in patients with surgically treated diabetic foot infection. J Foot Ankle Surg 2011;50:171–5.

22. Atway S, Nerone VS, Springer KD, et al. Rate of residual osteomyelitis after partial foot amputation in diabetic patients: a standardized method for evaluating bone margins with intraoperative culture. J Foot Ankle Surg 2012;51:749–52.

23. Fujii M, Terashi H, Yokono K. Surgical treatment strategy for diabetic forefoot osteomyelitis. Wound Repair Regen 2016;24:447–53.

24. Ruggiero SL, Dodson TB, Fantasia J, et al. American Association of Oral and Maxillofacial Surgeons position paper on medication-related osteonecrosis of the jaw–2014 update. J Oral Maxillofac Surg 2014; 72:1938–56.

25. Hamadeh IS, Ngwa BA, Gong Y. Drug induced osteonecrosis of the jaw. Cancer Treat Rev 2015;41: 455–64.

26. Diz P, López-Cedrún JL, Arenaz J, et al. Denosumab-related osteonecrosis of the jaw. J Am Dent Assoc 2012;143:981–4.

27. Ruggiero SL. Diagnosis and staging of medication-related osteonecrosis of the jaw. Oral Maxillofacial Surg Clin N Am 2015;27:479–87.

28. Epstein MS, Ephros HD, Epstein JB. Review of current literature and implications of RANKL inhibitors for oral health care providers. Oral Surg Oral Med Oral Pathol Oral Radiol 2013;116: e437–442.

29. Xu XL, Gou WL, Wang AY, et al. Basic research and clinical applications of bisphosphonates in bone disease: what have we learned over the last 40 years? J Transl Med 2013;11:303.

30. Aghaloo T, Hazboun R, Tetradis S. Pathophysiology of osteonecrosis of the jaws. Oral Maxillofacial Surg Clin N Am 2015;27:489–96.

31. Qaisi M, Hargett J, Loeb M, et al. Denosumab related osteonecrosis of the jaw with spontaneous necrosis of the soft palate: report of a life threatening case. Case Rep Dent 2016;2016:5070187.

32. Kajizono M, Sada H, Sugiura Y, et al. Incidence and risk factors of osteonecrosis of the jaw in advanced cancer patients after treatment with zoledronic acid or denosumab: a retrospective Cohort Study. Biol Pharm Bull 2015;38:1850–5.

33. Bamias A, Kastritis E, Bamia C, et al. Osteonecrosis of the jaw in cancer after treatment with bisphosphonates: incidence and risk factors. J Clin Oncol 2005;23:8580–7.

34. Khosla S, Burr D, Cauley J, et al. Bisphosphonate-associated osteonecrosis of the jaw: report of a task force of the American Society for Bone and Mineral Research. J Bone Miner Res 2007;22:1479–91.

35. Khan A. Osteonecrosis of the jaw: new developments in an old disease. J Rheumatol 2008;35: 547–9.

36. Marx RE, Sawatari Y, Fortin M, et al. Bisphosphonate-induced exposed bone (osteonecrosis/osteopetrosis) of the jaws: risk factors, recognition, prevention, and treatment. J Oral Maxillofac Surg 2005;63:1567–75.

37. Madrid C, Bouferrache K, Abarca M, et al. Bisphosphonate-related osteonecrosis of the jaws: how to manage cancer patients. Oral Oncol 2010; 46:468–70.

38. Bedogni A, Saia G, Bettini G, et al. Long-term outcomes of surgical resection of the jaws in cancer patients with bisphosphonate-related osteonecrosis. Oral Oncol 2011;47:420–4.

39. Carlson ER, Basile JD. The role of surgical resection in the management of bisphosphonate-related osteonecrosis of the jaws. J Oral Maxillofac Surg 2009;67(5 Suppl):85–95.

40. Bedogni A, Saia G, Ragazzo M, et al. Bisphosphonate-associated osteonecrosis can hide jaw metastases. Bone 2007;41:942–5.

41. Pautke C, Bauer F, Otto S, et al. Fluorescence-guided bone resection in bisphosphonate-related osteonecrosis of the jaws: first clinical results of a prospective pilot study. J Oral Maxillofac Surg 2011;69:84–91.

42. Ristow O, Pautke C. Auto-fluorescence of the bone and its use for delineation of bone necrosis. Int J Oral Maxillofac Surg 2014;43:1391–3.

43. Nocini PF, Saia G, Bettini G, et al. Vascularized fibula flap reconstruction of the mandible in bisphosphonate-related osteonecrosis. Eur J Surg Oncol 2009;35:373–9.

44. Bedogni A, Blandamura S, Lokmic Z, et al. Bisphosphonate-associated jawbone osteonecrosis: a correlation between imaging techniques and histopathology. Oral Surg Oral Med Oral Pathol Oral Radiol Endod 2008;105:358–64.

45. Cho YA, Yoon HJ, Lee JI, et al. Histopathological features of bisphosphonate-associated osteonecrosis: findings in patients treated with partial mandibulectomies. Oral Surg Oral Med Oral Pathol Oral Radiol 2012;114:785–91.

46. Hansen T, Kunkel M, Weber A, et al. Osteonecrosis of the jaws in patients treated with bisphosphonates: histomorphologic analysis in comparison with infected osteoradionecrosis. J Oral Pathol Med 2006;35:155–60.

47. Carlson ER, Fleisher KE, Ruggiero SL. Metastatic cancer identified in osteonecrosis specimens of the jaws in patients receiving intravenous bisphosphonate medications. J Oral Maxillofac Surg 2013;71:2077–86.

48. Shaw RJ, Dhanda J. Hyperbaric oxygen in the management of late radiation injury to the head and neck. Part I: treatment. Br J Oral Maxillofac Surg 2011;49:2–8.

49. Støre G, Boysen M. Mandibular osteoradionecrosis: clinical behaviour and diagnostic aspects. Clin Otolaryngol Allied Sci 2000;25:378–84.

50. Chopra S, Kamdar D, Ugur OE, et al. Factors predictive of severity of osteoradionecrosis of the mandible. Head Neck 2011;33:1600–5.

51. Marx RE. Osteoradionecrosis: a new concept of its pathophysiology. J Oral Maxillofac Surg 1983;41: 283–8.

52. Thorn JJ, Hansen HS, Specht L, et al. Osteoradionecrosis of the jaws: clinical characteristics and relation to the field of irradiation. J Oral Maxillofac Surg 2000;58:1088–93 [discussion: 1093–5].

53. Gevorgyan A, Wong K, Poon I, et al. Osteoradionecrosis of the mandible: a case series at a single institution. J Otolaryngol Head Neck Surg 2013;42:46.

54. Ben-David MA, Diamante M, Radawski JD, et al. Lack of osteoradionecrosis of the mandible after intensity-modulated radiotherapy for head and neck cancer: likely contributions of both dental care and improved dose distributions. Int J Radiat Oncol Biol Phys 2007;68:396–402.

55. Gomez DR, Estilo CL, Wolden SL, et al. Correlation of osteoradionecrosis and dental events with dosimetric parameters in intensity-modulated radiation therapy for head-and-neck cancer. Int J Radiat Oncol Biol Phys 2011;81:e207–213.

56. Peterson DE, Doerr W, Hovan A, et al. Osteoradionecrosis in cancer patients: the evidence base for treatment-dependent frequency, current management

strategies, and future studies. Support Care Cancer 2010;18:1089–98.

57. Lyons A, Ghazali N. Osteoradionecrosis of the jaws: current understanding of its pathophysiology and treatment. Br J Oral Maxillofac Surg 2008;46: 653–60.

58. Notani K, Yamazaki Y, Kitada H, et al. Management of mandibular osteoradionecrosis corresponding to the severity of osteoradionecrosis and the method of radiotherapy. Head Neck 2003;25:181–6.

59. Tibbles PM, Edelsberg JS. Hyperbaric-oxygen therapy. N Engl J Med 1996;334:1642–8.

60. Annane D, Depondt J, Aubert P, et al. Hyperbaric oxygen therapy for radionecrosis of the jaw: a randomized, placebo-controlled, double-blind trial from the ORN96 study group. J Clin Oncol 2004; 22:4893–900.

61. Marx RE, Johnson RP, Kline SN. Prevention of osteoradionecrosis: a randomized prospective clinical trial of hyperbaric oxygen versus penicillin. J Am Dent Assoc 1985;111:49–54.

62. Marx RE, Ehler WJ, Tayapongsak P, et al. Relationship of oxygen dose to angiogenesis induction in irradiated tissue. Am J Surg 1990;160:519–24.

63. Lubek JE, Hancock MK, Strome SE. What is the value of hyperbaric oxygen therapy in management of osteoradionecrosis of the head and neck? Laryngoscope 2013;123:555–6.

64. Gal TJ, Yueh B, Futran ND. Influence of prior hyperbaric oxygen therapy in complications following microvascular reconstruction for advanced osteoradionecrosis. Arch Otolaryngol Head Neck Surg 2003;129:72–6.

65. Delanian S, Depondt J, Lefaix JL. Major healing of refractory mandible osteoradionecrosis after treatment combining pentoxifylline and tocopherol: a phase II trial. Head Neck 2005;27:114–23.

66. Delanian S, Chatel C, Porcher R, et al. Complete restoration of refractory mandibular osteoradionecrosis by prolonged treatment with a pentoxifylline-tocopherol-clodronate combination (PENTOCLO): a phase II trial. Int J Radiat Oncol Biol Phys 2011;80: 832–9.

67. Curi MM, Oliveira dos Santos M, Feher O, et al. Management of extensive osteoradionecrosis of the mandible with radical resection and immediate microvascular reconstruction. J Oral Maxillofac Surg 2007;65:434–8.

68. Chang DW, Oh HK, Robb GL, et al. Management of advanced mandibular osteoradionecrosis with free flap reconstruction. Head Neck 2001;23:830–5.

69. Alam DS, Nuara M, Christian J. Analysis of outcomes of vascularized flap reconstruction in patients with advanced mandibular osteoradionecrosis. Otolaryngol Head Neck Surg 2009;141:196–201.

70. Hirsch DL, Bell RB, Dierks EJ, et al. Analysis of microvascular free flaps for reconstruction of advanced mandibular osteoradionecrosis: a retrospective cohort study. J Oral Maxillofac Surg 2008; 66:2545–56.

71. Suh JD, Blackwell KE, Sercarz JA, et al. Disease relapse after segmental resection and free flap reconstruction for mandibular osteoradionecrosis. Otolaryngol Head Neck Surg 2010;142:586–91.

72. Zaghi S, Miller M, Blackwell K, et al. Analysis of surgical margins in cases of mandibular osteoradionecrosis that progress despite extensive mandible resection and free tissue transfer. Am J Otolaryngol 2012;33:576–80.

73. Maurer P, Meyer L. Osteoradionecrosis of the mandible–Resection aided by measurement of partial pressure of oxygen (pO2): a technical report. J Oral Maxillofac Surg 2006;64:560–2.

74. Pautke C, Bauer F, Bissinger O, et al. Tetracycline bone fluorescence: a valuable marker for osteonecrosis characterization and therapy. J Oral Maxillofac Surg 2010;68:125–9.

75. Schilling C, Ahmed N, Jayaram R, et al. Intraoperative assessment of osteoradionecrosis (ORN) affected tissue by near infrared (NIR) fluorescence imaging [abstract]. Br J Oral Maxillofac Surg 2015; e114.

76. Hansen T, Kunkel M, Springer E, et al. Actinomycosis of the jaws–histopathological study of 45 patients shows significant involvement in bisphosphonate-associated osteonecrosis and infected osteoradionecrosis. Virchows Arch 2007;451:1009–17.

77. Marwan H, Green JM, Tursun R, et al. Recurrent malignancy in osteoradionecrosis specimen. J Oral Maxillofac Surg 2016;74:2312–6.

Margin Analysis
Malignant Salivary Gland Neoplasms of the Head and Neck

Robert A. Ord, MS, MBA, FRCS[a],*,
Naseem Ghazali, MSc, DOHNS, FDSRCS, FRCS(ÖMFS)[b]

KEYWORDS

- Salivary gland • Cancer • Malignancy • Surgical margins

KEY POINTS

- Surgical margins are dependent on histology and grade.
- The facial nerve is preserved unless infiltrated/encased.
- Palatal bone is preserved in low-grade mucoepidermoid carcinoma unless it is clinically/radiologically invaded.
- In adenoid cystic carcinoma, involved major nerves should be traced and have frozen section sampling.

INTRODUCTION

Most definitions of negative surgical margins in oncologic surgery are based on the histopathologic specimen and state that a mandatory minimum distance between ink and tumor is necessary for good local control. A minimum effective margin is the ideal because excising more tissue may not give any increased local control and adds more morbidity. Even in the common head and neck cancers (eg, squamous cell carcinomas), controversy exists in what constitutes a negative margin. The protocols for margins in salivary gland cancer are not well established for several reasons.

Salivary gland malignancies are rare, comprising 3% of head and neck cancers, which are only 3% of all cancers. This means there are few large series and an absence of prospective randomized trials. The paucity of evidence-based data to help establish the correct distance for a surgical margin in salivary cancer (SC) is further compounded by the different sites involved by these tumors and their diverse histologic types. There is not a single identifiable margin for all tumor types and sites because some of these entities are represented in the literature by only a small number of case reports. To try and rationalize this topic, paranasal sinus, tracheal, laryngeal, and oropharyngeal minor salivary gland tumors are not discussed. Submandibular and sublingual gland tumors are not analyzed in depth other than as major salivary gland tumors. Rare histologic subtypes (eg, cystadenocarcinoma, sclerosing clear cell carcinoma) are also not included. This article concentrates on trying to establish, from the literature, what is an acceptable surgical margin for the more common SCs, found in the minor salivary glands of the oral cavity and the parotid gland.

The data from a large series of SCs of the parotid and major salivary glands suggest that prognosis is related to TNM staging and histologic

Disclaimer: The authors have no conflict of interest, including any financial or funding sources, to declare.
[a] Department of Oral and Maxillofacial Surgery, University of Maryland Dental School, University of Maryland Medical Center, Greenebaum Cancer Center, Suite 1401, 650, West Baltimore Street, Baltimore, MD 21201, USA; [b] Oncology/Microvascular Surgery, University of Maryland Dental School, University of Maryland Medical Center, Greenbaum Cancer Center, Suite 1401, 650, West Baltimore Street, Baltimore, MD 21201, USA
* Corresponding author.
E-mail address: rord@umm.edu

differentiation.[1] In other series additional prognostic factors included are extraglandular extension, aggressive histology, facial nerve involvement, and advancing age.[2–4]

None of these authors mentions margin status as a prognostic factor. However, data from fast neutron analysis show that advanced SC with gross residual disease has a 6-year local-regional control of 59% but 100% if there is no evidence of residual disease,[5] so that evidently complete tumor resection and margin status must have a prognostic role in SC. A recent study on 301 cases from Memorial Sloan Kettering hospital developed postoperative nomograms to predict survival for major gland SC.[6] The authors found the five variables associated with predicting cancer-specific survival were (1) histologic grade, (2) perineural invasion, (3) clinical T4, (4) positive node status, and (5) status of margins (confidence interval, 0.856). In a national review of SC in Denmark with 871 cases of major and minor SC, microscopic margins were an independent prognostic factor for crude and disease specific survival (DSS) in multivariate analysis, and independent prognostic factor for recurrence-free survival. Involved or close microscopic margins were also independent prognostic factors with a negative impact on survival.[7]

Given that there are a large number of histologic types of SC this article broadly classifies tumors into low-grade and high-grade. There are some tumor types that do not fall into these categories easily and adenoid cystic carcinoma (ACC) and carcinoma ex pleomorphic adenoma (CExPA) are reviewed as separate entities.

SITE-SPECIFIC CONSIDERATIONS

In the parotid the surgeon is constrained by the management of the facial nerve. Most surgeons attempt to preserve the facial nerve unless it is infiltrated or embedded in the tumor making sacrifice inevitable.[8,9] There is little evidence to show improved survival with facial nerve sacrifice and adjuvant radiation can give local control. Even with nerve sacrifice and adjuvant radiation patients with preoperative facial palsy had only a 13% disease-free survival compared with 69% in those patients with a normally functioning nerve.[10] A recent retrospective study of 129 patients showed disease recurrence in 64% of patients with both facial nerve palsy and perineural infiltration, 43% in patients with only facial nerve palsy, 27% with only perineural infiltration, and 16% in patients with neither.[11] In a series of patients with parotid cancer who had no preoperative facial nerve palsy and underwent nerve-sparing surgery, survival rates were better than the patients who had nerve

sacrifice.[12] Most studies support the idea of preserving the facial nerve whenever possible and that in most cases there is little improvement of outcome with sacrificing the nerve.

In the oral cavity, the most common site for minor salivary tumors is the posterior hard palate. In these cases consideration must be given to the bone margin and whether palatal fenestration or maxillectomy is essential. It is also important for the pathologist to realize that a tumor invading the floor of the sinus may involve the sinus lining but that this is not a positive margin but a "surgical margin." In this case the sinus cavity is the next "barrier" so the margin is not close to any anatomic structure. Additionally, the greater palatine nerve may be a pathway to the skull base for neurotropic tumors.

LOW-GRADE SALIVARY MALIGNANCIES

In examining margins for low-grade salivary malignancies, we consider low-grade mucoepidermoid carcinoma (LGMEC), acinic cell carcinoma, and low-grade polymorphous adenocarcinoma (LGPA).

LGMEC is the most common SC in oral minor salivary tumors and in the parotid, whereas acinic cell carcinoma is the third most common SC with greater than 80% involving the parotid.[13] They are both slow growing and rarely metastasize. One series of mucoepidermoid carcinomas (MECs) of the parotid from the Mayo Clinic showed 98.9% 5-year, 97.4% 10-year, and 97.4% 25-year survival in T1/2 lesions (83 of 89 cases low or intermediate grade).[14] Certainly in relation to the parotid gland a parotidectomy with a cuff of 5 mm of normal parotid tissue is sufficient margin for all but large T4 tumors. Even when the tumor abuts the facial nerve it should not be sacrificed and capsular dissection should give an adequate margin if there is no infiltration of the nerve (**Fig. 1**). Evidence for this statement is provided by McGurk and coworkers.[15] In this retrospective study of 662 parotid tumors (<4 cm, clinically benign), 503 patients underwent extracapsular dissection (ECD). Twelve cases were malignant on final pathology having had the ECD, but the 5- and 10-year survival rates were 100%. In this cohort of 12 patients, there were seven LGMECs and a single case of acinic cell carcinoma. There was one local recurrence (a papillary adenocarcinoma) and seven of the cases had radiotherapy for either positive margins or high-grade histology. The authors concluded that ECD was a viable alternative to superficial parotidectomy for most parotid tumors without oncologic compromise and giving less morbidity.

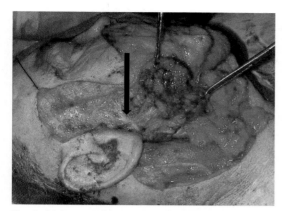

Fig. 1. Right parotidectomy and selective neck dissection for low-grade SC. The facial nerve can be preserved (*black arrow*).

Despite the excellent prognosis of these types of parotid tumors, caution should be taken with acinic cell carcinomas that are greater than 3 cm in men and patients older than 45 years, to maximize local control.[16] Again in LGMEC advanced stage, perineural invasion, submandibular gland location, and positive margins all predict poor outcome, although intermediate grade has the same favorable survival as the low grade.[17] In cases with positive margins reresection may be possible, but if the margin is against the facial nerve studies have shown excellent local control with minimal morbidity for post-operative radiation for small LGMEC and acinic cell carcinoma of the parotid with positive margins.[18]

In minor salivary gland tumors of the oral cavity, acinic cell carcinomas are rare. In the author's unpublished series of 300 cases only four were acinic cell carcinoma. LGMEC and intermediate-grade MECs are the most common SC in the oral cavity and represent 45.5% of all malignant tumors in the author's series. The most common site is the palate, at 42%. Although the author prefers an 8-to-10-mm soft tissue margin around the palpable tumor there is controversy regarding whether the underlying bone of the hard palate should be resected. Usually theses tumors are discovered when less than 2 cm and with no clinical or radiologic evidence of bone involvement. In these situations for squamous cell carcinoma (a high-grade cancer) overlying the mandible it is generally accepted that if periosteal stripping does not show penetration of the periosteum or cortical bone involvement the mandible need not be resected even if the margin is only a few millimeters.[19] Eversole and colleagues[20] first reported this approach for LGMEC in 1972 in low- and intermediate-grade MECs without bone erosion

with 100% cure. This was supported by a study on 54 intraoral MECs, which also recommended that well-differentiated tumors behaved benignly and are best treated by modest local excision without jaw excision.[21] A dissenting study from the Mayo Clinic also with 54 cases of intraoral MEC recommended partial maxillectomy irrespective of stage or grade.

In a previous study by the current author (RAO), 18 patients had low/intermediate T1 MECs of the palate, 16 of which were treated by palatal periosteal stripping. Eleven patients had clear margins, three had less than 1 mm deep margin, and two had invasion of the periosteal margin. No local recurrence was found in any of our cohort and the follow-up average time for the close/positive margin patients was 61 months.[22] The authors' now have 39 patients with T1 low/intermediate grade MEC of the palate, only four of which have required bone resection (**Fig. 2**) and the rest treated with periosteal stripping, and they continue to have zero recurrence for palatal tumors (Ord RA, unpublished data, 2017) (**Fig. 3**).

LGPA has excellent reported survival and the palate is the most common site. In 164 cases treated with surgery only, 97.6% were alive at an average of 115.4 months follow-up.[23] In another SEER data review of 460 cases (2001–2011) 10-year DSS was 96.4% and 57.2% of tumors were palatal.[24] However, despite this excellent survival and rare occurrence of regional and distant metastases LGPA requires complete resection. In a case series and extensive literature review Kimple and colleagues[25] identified 456 cases with an overall local recurrence of 19%. Half the recurrences appeared by 36 months but the range extended to 24 years. The authors recommend wide local excision.[25] The previously mentioned studies do not show that radiation is necessarily effective as an adjuvant therapy and has worse survival used as a single prime therapy so that effective primary surgery is essential. Some authors have proposed that because some LGPA may show clinical behavior that is not low grade, they should be called polymorphous adenocarcinoma.[26] Certainly a 1-cm soft tissue margin should be used and this author believes that bone removal is required even when there is no direct invasion. These tumors also show a high rate of perineural involvement, which does not seem to carry the same poor prognostic value as that seen in ACC. Despite its low-grade classification and excellent survival outcome local recurrence is a higher risk than for LGMEC or acinic cell carcinoma.

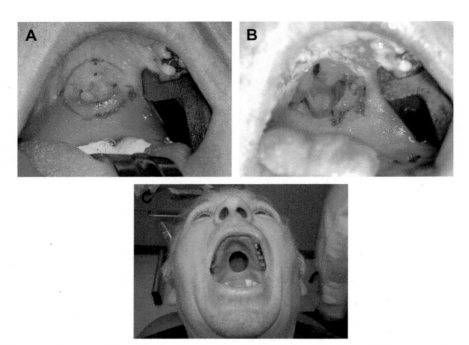

Fig. 2. (*A*) Low-grade mucoepidermoid carcinoma of the hard palate with 1-cm soft tissue margin marked out before incision. (*B*) At the time of surgery the bone was found to be invaded and was resected along with the nasal lining. (*C*) Six months postoperative shows defect before delayed reconstruction with a microvascular radial forearm flap.

POTENTIALLY AGGRESSIVE SALIVARY MALIGNANCIES

The following discussion is limited to two tumors that may show features of both high- and low-grade SC the ACC and the CExPA.

ACC is a cancer that has many features of a low-grade tumor. Being slow growing with a low mitotic rate, it rarely metastasizes to regional nodes and has an excellent 5-year survival rate. However, it does show a high rate of local recurrence and relentless progression, with eventual blood-borne metastases to lung, liver, and bone with a 10-to-20-year survival that is, comparable with a high-grade tumor. The survival and prognosis are related to stage, perineural invasion, and histologic type (tubular, cribriform, or solid). The ACC is found in major and minor salivary glands, but more in the minor glands. In the parotid gland involvement and invasion of the nerve may involve wide resection of the nerve including temporal bone dissection because of the ability of the ACC to display perineural invasion and travel along the nerve (**Fig. 4**).

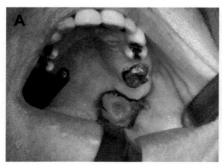
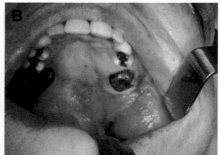

Fig. 3. (*A*) Low-grade mucoepidermoid carcinoma of the left posterior palate marked with a 1-cm soft tissue margin before incision. (*B*) Bone was uninvolved when the periosteum was lifted off the palate so the palatal bone was preserved and reconstruction of the defect is with a buccal fat pad flap.

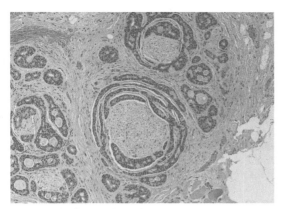

Fig. 4. Cribriform adenoid cystic carcinoma showing perineural invasion (hematoxilin and eosin).

In 1986, Matsuba and colleagues[27] showed that perineural spread occurred in 33% to 85% of cases and that 5-year survival and local recurrence were 93.8% and 26.7% without perineural spread but 36.9% and 81.8%, respectively, with perineural spread. The authors showed a 0% of distant metastases with negative surgical margins and no perineural spread, but a 40% incidence of distant metastases when both these factors were present. This paper also highlighted the poor prognosis for solid-type ACC followed by cribriform. This classic study did emphasize the poor prognosis related to perineural spread. However, perineural invasion is more likely as the ACC increases in size and other authors have believed that perhaps size is the more important variable. In one recent retrospective study with 26 cases there was no correlation between perineural invasion and size of the primary tumor, positive surgical margins, distant metastases, or local control.[28] However, perineural invasion was associated with local extension and outcome. Their literature review showed perineural invasion in 15% to 72% of cases of ACC and local recurrence in 13% to 52%. In a large series of 105 cases the 5-, 10-, and 20-year survival rates were 68%, 52%, and 28% with stage, grade, age, and surgical margins being the main predictors of survival.[29]

The high rates of positive margins and local recurrence seen in most series are associated with deceptive, widespread local infiltration and the ability of the tumor to travel along nerves via the perineural spaces (**Fig. 5**). This mandates generous soft tissue margins 1.5 to 2 cm where possible and excision of bone with maxillectomy for palatal tumors. Frozen section guidance is

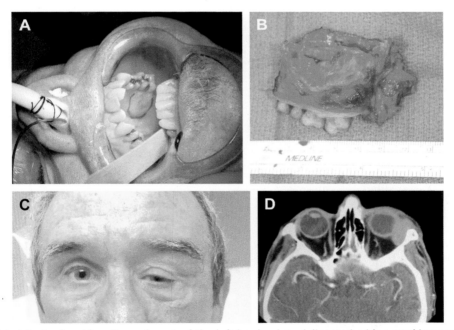

Fig. 5. (A) Indolent adenoid cystic carcinoma of the left hard palate delineated with a marking pen to better demonstrate the extent of palpable tumor before maxillectomy with 1.5-cm margins. (B) Maxillectomy specimen through the left canine socket and including pterygoid plates. The greater palatine nerve showed involvement and was traced superiorly. The patient had postoperative radiation therapy. (C) Nine months postsurgery the patient presents with lacrimal gland swelling and ptosis. (D) Computed tomography shows metastatic adenoid cystic carcinoma in the lacrimal gland from perineural spread.

helpful for the soft tissue margins and for any major nerve that may be involved (eg, the greater palatine nerve) to try and ensure the margin is negative. Unfortunately, the perineural spread may show skip lesions beyond a region of the nerve that is clinically negative, and spread may be a considerable distance beyond the primary tumor (**Fig. 6**). These lesions are challenging to ensure surgical clearance and their slow rate of growth may mean that local recurrence may be delayed many years. It does seem that adjuvant radiation therapy may improve local control.

CExPA is also a salivary malignancy with uncertain behavior, which occurs mostly in the parotid and major glands. Unlike squamous cell carcinoma of the oral cavity salivary gland cancers usually arise *de novo* without a preceding benign or premalignant lesion being present. The exception is the CexPA, which arises in a benign pleomorphic adenoma usually of greater than 10 years and the malignant change is presumed secondary to accumulated genetic mutations. When planning surgical management and margins there are two considerations; the histologic type of malignancy (low or high grade) and the relationship of the cancer to the capsule of the pleomorphic adenoma.

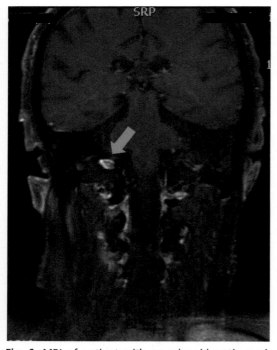

Fig. 6. MRI of patient with an adenoid cystic carcinoma in the right palate. In the coronal view, there is enhancement in the right pterygopalatine fossa caused by tumor involvement (*arrow*). The right vidian canal also showed abnormal enhancement.

Generally the malignant change seen is high grade and these tumors are regarded as aggressive requiring wide local excision, neck dissection, and possible adjuvant radiation. However, low-grade malignant can be treated less radically.

The World Health Organization subclassifies CExPA based on capsular invasion into noninvasive, minimally invasive (<1.5 mm penetration of the malignant component into the extracapsular tissue), and invasive (>1.5 mm of invasion from the tumor capsule into adjacent tissues).[30] This differentiation is important because noninvasive (also called carcinoma in situ arising in a pleomorphic adenoma) and minimally invasive tumors have an excellent prognosis. In these cases surgical margins can be conservative, with a few millimeters or even ECD for noninvasive and 5 to 10 mm for minimally invasive tumors. The exception may be tumors that show myoepithelial carcinomas, which show a greater risk of recurrence and metastasis even in noninvasive and minimally invasive tumors.[31] Other authors have questioned the World Health Organization classification in terms of measured invasion, stating that the threshold for distinguishing capsular invasion with good prognosis from poor prognosis is 5 mm and that cases greater than 8 mm do poorly.[32] Griffith and colleagues[33] showed most (61%) CExPA were widely invasive at presentation, only 11.4% were noninvasive, and their cutoff threshold for good prognosis was 2 mm of extracapsular invasion. A further study of 58 cases showed there were no metastases or deaths in tumors less than 2.5 mm invasion; however, 13 of their cases with invasion exceeding 2.5 mm did well confirming that it is not just invasiveness that decides outcome.[34]

HIGH-GRADE MALIGNANCIES

Histologic types of salivary carcinomas that are considered biologically aggressive or high-grade malignancy include CExPA, salivary duct carcinoma (SDC), carcinosarcoma (malignant mixed tumor), squamous cell carcinoma, oncocytic carcinoma, and small and large cell carcinoma. Other SC can demonstrate a range of biologic behavior within a histologic type. Grading may further identify subgroups within the principle histologic type, such as in MEC, adenocarcinoma not otherwise specified (NOS), and ACC. In addition, high-grade versions of intrinsically low-grade tumors can also exist *de novo* (eg, the papillary cystic variant of acinic cell carcinoma) or develop from high-grade transformation of low-grade tumors.[35,36]

High-grade salivary carcinoma is associated with a high-risk of treatment failure, prompting an aggressive, multimodality approach. Standard management of surgically resectable high-grade carcinomas of the major and minor salivary glands includes surgical excision of the primary site and neck dissection.[37] A selective prophylactic neck dissection is considered appropriate, and when there is evidence of nodal involvement, conventional neck dissection forms part of standard treatment. Postoperative adjuvant radiation is recommended in high-grade salivary carcinoma and in cases of close or positive margins. Other circumstances warranting postoperative radiation are presence of perineural invasion, presence of advanced disease (eg, involvement of facial nerve/deep parotid lobe), and/or lymphovascular invasion. The rarity of high-grade salivary malignancy makes it challenging to obtain robust evidence in ascertaining the impact of using these high-risk variables on treatment outcomes when used in treatment decision-making for adjuvant radiotherapy. It is under this context that the discussion on margin status is henceforth considered.

Because ACC and CExPA are considered in a separate section, the following discussion focuses mainly on high-grade MEC and SDC, where there is sufficient published evidence to draw limited conclusions regarding the status of margins. Although there are small studies that show margins are a prognostic indicator for adenocarcinoma NOS, sebaceous carcinoma, and mucinous adenocarcinoma, there are too few series to provide any real guidelines.

High-grade MEC are generally treated with surgical excision with wide margins followed by postoperative radiotherapy. Neck dissection is often used when regional metastasis is present. Frequency of close and/or involved margins for low, intermediate or high grade tumor is 5% to 11%, 13.8% to 22%, and 33% to 72%, respectively,[38–43] with a trend toward lower rates of positive margins in studies with higher proportion of cases where the primary site was oral cavity/minor salivary gland sites.

Most MEC studies report treatment outcomes as an overall group, where high-grade and nodal involvement are the most common predictive factors of outcome.[44,45] There is less uniform finding in regard to resection margin status. In some MEC studies, resection margin status prognosticates survival outcomes but not in others.[42,46,47] In addition, resection margins may be a predictor on univariate analysis but not on multivariate analysis. Fewer studies consider subgroup analysis of outcomes based on grading. In one study, positive surgical margin was a significant predictor for poorer disease-free survival in high-grade MEC subtypes and forms the rationale for recommending wide surgical excision of the primary lesion with particular emphasis on obtaining negative surgical margins to avoid local recurrence.[42] Postoperative radiotherapy augmented locoregional control when positive resection margins were present.

SDC is rare (1%–3% of all salivary carcinomas), and represents an aggressive salivary gland carcinoma with poor prognosis, which histologically resembles high-grade ductal breast carcinoma. Surgical approaches to the primary site frequently involve wide local resection, and because SDC most commonly occurs in major glands (93%–100%), the entire gland is removed. Despite its aggressive clinical behavior, some advocate for "conservative" resections (ie, partial parotidectomy with nerve preservation), particularly for tumors less than 2 cm isolated to the superficial aspect of the parotid gland where nerve function was normal preoperatively, because more radical treatment has not shown significant survival benefit.[48] Presence of facial palsy is considered a surrogate marker of nerve involvement by tumor preoperatively, and facial nerve sacrifice is usually undertaken during surgery. Variations of radical parotidectomy are performed with different degrees of nerve sacrifice to obtain oncologic clearance. Facial nerve margin status is not often reported even though it may be associated with local recurrence. In a large series from a single institution, and 9 of 54 local failures (17%) occurred where the primary tumor was located in the parotid (eight cases) and submandibular (one case).[49] A total of 75% of patients with parotid recurrence presented with facial nerve paresis/paralysis and nerve involvement by tumor at or proximal to the styloid foramen. In this cohort, the reported positive facial nerve margin was 60% but the local recurrence numbers were too small for any meaningful statistical analysis for its predictive value.

Even with a radical surgical approach, achieving microscopically negative surgical margins is challenging.[50] Overall, the reported positive resection margin rates for SDC are 9% to 66% (mean, 41.6%). The impact of involved surgical margin in survival outcomes is not fully established. This variable is not always included in univariate and multivariate analyses in SDC studies that report it. A nationwide Danish study based on cancer registry data (n = 34) found that involved margins were predictors of overall survival and 5-year disease-free survival on multivariate analysis.[51] Other SDC studies report an association between margin status with overall survival,[52] progression-free survival,[53] and distant metastasis–free survival on univariate analysis[54]

Adjuvant radiotherapy provides an additional means to obtain locoregional control postoperatively, particularly in the presence of involved surgical margins and positive nodal status. Additional radiation dose is given to the surgical bed with a positive surgical margin. The clinical target volume is extended to the base of skull when a named (cranial) nerve margin is positive.[55] However, the overall impact of adjuvant radiotherapy on outcomes remains debatable,[56] in light of high locoregional and distant recurrence rates, and unclear survival benefit.

CENTRAL (INTRAOSSEOUS) SALIVARY GLAND CARCINOMA

Central malignant salivary gland tumors of the jaw are rare, constituting less than 0.4% of all salivary gland carcinomas.[57] The two histologic types most commonly found are MEC (most common) and ACC. Surgical treatment of central salivary gland malignancy has ranged from enucleation or curettage to en bloc or radical resection. More recently, these rare tumors are addressed with aggressive surgical resection (ie, wide local resection)[58–62] because higher local recurrence rates are seen with enucleation/curettage (40%–45%) than resection (13%). Varying degrees of mandibulectomy and maxillectomy are performed depending on the desired clear surgical margin to be achieved, especially in context of the mandible. The authors have usually treated these tumors like ameloblastomas because most are LGMECs with 1-cm margins and resection of at least one anatomic barrier of soft tissue if the cortical plate is perforated. Neck dissection is performed for clinically positive nodal status and the author undertakes supraomohyoid neck dissection for N0 disease. This is because there has been a high incidence of occult disease in our small series (23.5% for retromolar fossa and intraosseous LGMEC) and the neck is entered anyway as the cervical approach to segmental mandibulectomy. Prognosis is difficult to determine with certainly because of the rarity of this condition and the varying range of treatment administered. It is suggested that a better prognosis tends to be seen with well-differentiated, low-grade tumor without perineural invasion and with tumor-free margin.

Resection margin status was not always reported. Clean surgical margins are more challenging to obtain in more advanced tumors especially when cortical plates have been breached. In the maxilla, extension beyond the confines of the jaw into soft tissues and the pterygoid plates makes it difficult to obtain clear surgical margins even with total maxillectomy.

SUMMARY

The rarity of salivary carcinomas, the diversity of histologic types, and the differing behavior at its different sites make it difficult to form evidence-based conclusions regarding what are the best oncologic margins for these tumors. Certainly low-grade SC can usually be treated with 1-cm margins and the facial nerve is preserved in parotidectomy unless clinically involved. In palatal LGMEC the authors believe that bone resection is not indicated unless there is clinical/radiologic evidence of invasion. The margin necessary for CexPA depends on the status of the tumor in relation to the capsule, and for tumors that are intracapsular or less than 2 mm outside the capsule a conservative resection is usually sufficient.

In the case of ACC wide margins of at least 1.5 cm where possible are required with frozen section analysis. Any involved nerves should be traced proximally and clearance assessed by frozen section. In many of the high-grade tumors there is insufficient evidence to give good guidelines so that these tumors are usually treated like squamous cell carcinomas with minimum margins of 1 cm clinically and regarding a final surgical histologic margin of less than 5 mm as "close" and possibly requiring adjuvant radiotherapy.

Intraosseous tumors are usually low-grade and are removed using the same criteria for margins as ameloblastoma.

REFERENCES

1. Harbo G, Bungaard T, Pedersen D, et al. Prognostic indicators for malignant tumors of the parotid gland. Clin Otolaryngol Allied Sci 2002;27(6):512–6.
2. Hocwald E, Korkmaz H, Yoo GH, et al. Prognostic factors in major salivary gland cancer. Laryngoscope 2001;111(8):1434–9.
3. Lima RA, Tavares MR, Dias FL, et al. Clinical prognostic factors in malignant parotid tumors. Otolaryngol Head Neck Surg 2005;133:702–8.
4. Bhattacharyya N, Fried MP. Determinants of survival in parotid cancer: a population based study. Am J Otolaryngol 2005;26:39–44.
5. Douglas JG, Koh WJ, Austin-Seymour M, et al. Treatment of salivary gland neoplasms with fast neutron radiotherapy. Arch Otolaryngol Head Neck Surg 2003;129:944–8.
6. Ali S, Palmer FL, Yu C, et al. Postoperative nomograms predictive of survival after surgical management of malignant tumors of the major salivary glands. Ann Surg Oncol 2014;21(2):637–42.
7. Bjørndal K, Krogdahl A, Therkildsen MH, et al. Salivary gland carcinoma in Denmark 1990-2005: outcome and prognostic factors. Results of the

Danish Head and Neck Cancer Group (DAHANCA). Oral Oncol 2012;48(2):179–85.

8. Spiro JD, Spiro RH. Cancer of the parotid gland: role of 7th nerve preservation. World J Surg 2003;27(7):863–7.

9. Carinci F, Farina A, Pelucchi S, et al. Parotid gland carcinoma: surgical strategy based on local risk factors. J Craniofac Surg 2001;12(5):434–7.

10. Terhaard C, Lubsen H, Tan B, et al. Facial nerve function in carcinoma of the parotid gland. Eur J Cancer 2006;42(16):2744–50.

11. Terakedis BE, Hunt JP, Buchmann LO, et al. The prognostic significance of facial nerve involvement in carcinomas of the parotid gland. Am J Clin Oncol 2014. [Epub ahead of print].

12. Guntinas-Lichius O, Klussman JP, Schroeder U, et al. Primary parotid malignant surgery in patients with normal preoperative facial nerve function: outcome and long-term postoperative facial nerve function. Laryngoscope 2004;114(5):949–56.

13. Ellis GL, Auclair P. Tumors of the salivary glands. Atlas of tumor pathology. 4th series. Fascicle 9. Washington, DC: Armed Forces Institute of Pathology; 2008. p. 368–72.

14. Boahene DK, Olsen KD, Lewis JE, et al. Mucoepidermoid carcinoma of the parotid gland: the Mayo clinic experience. Arch Otolaryngol Head Neck Surg 2004;130(7):849–56.

15. McGurk M, Thomas BL, Renehan AG. Extracapsular dissection for clinically benign parotid lumps: reduced morbidity without oncological compromise. Br J Cancer 2003;89(9):1610–3.

16. Neskey DM, Klein JD, Hicks S, et al. Prognostic factors associated with decreased survival in patients with acinic cell carcinoma. JAMA Otolaryngol Head Neck Surg 2013;139(11):1195–202.

17. McHugh CH, Roberts DB, El-Naggar AK, et al. Prognostic factors in mucoepidermoid carcinoma of the salivary glands. JAMA Otolaryngol Head Neck Surg 2013;139(11):1195–202.

18. Richter SM, Friedmann P, Mourad WF, et al. Postoperative radiation therapy for small, low-/intermediate-grade parotid tumors with close and/or positive surgical margins. Head Neck 2012;34(7):953–5.

19. Brown JS, Lewis-Jones H. Evidence for imaging the mandible in the management of oral squamous cell carcinoma: a review. Br J Oral Maxillofac Surg 2001; 39:411–8.

20. Eversole LR, Rovin S, Sabes WR. Mucoepidermoid carcinoma of minor salivary glands: report of 17 cases with follow-up. J Oral Surg 1972;30:107–12.

21. Melrose RJ, Abram AM, Howell FV. Mucoepidermoid tumors of the intraoral minor salivary glands: a clinicopathologic study of 54 cases. J Oral Pathol 1973;2:314–25.

22. Ord RA, Salama AR. Is it necessary to resect bone for low-grade mucoepidermoid carcinoma of the palate? Br J Oral Maxillofac Surg 2012;50(8):712–4.

23. Castle JT, Thompson LD, Frommelt RA, et al. Polymorphous low-grade adenocarcinoma: a clinicopathologic study of 164 cases. Cancer 1999;86(2): 207–19.

24. Patel TD, Vazquez A, Marchiano E, et al. Polymorphous low-grade adenocarcinoma of the head and neck: a population-based study of 460 cases. Laryngoscope 2015;125(7):1644–9.

25. Kimple AJ, Austin GK, Shah RN, et al. Polymorphous low-grade adenocarcinoma: a case series and determination of recurrence. Laryngoscope 2014; 124(12):2714–9.

26. Speight PM, Barrett AW. Salivary gland tumors. Oral Dis 2002;8(5):229–40.

27. Matsuba HM, Spector GJ, Thawley SE, et al. Adenoid cystic salivary gland carcinoma. A histopathologic review of treatment failure patterns. Cancer 1986;57(3):519–24.

28. Lukšić I, Suton P, Macan D, et al. Intraoral adenoid cystic carcinoma: is the presence of perineural invasion associated with the size of the primary tumour, local extension, surgical margins, distant metastases and outcome? Br J Oral Maxfac Surg 2014;52: 214–8.

29. van Weert S, Bloemena E, van der Waal I, et al. Adenoid cystic carcinoma of the head and neck: a single-center analysis of 105 consecutive cases over a 30-year period. Oral Oncol 2013;49(8):824–9.

30. Gnepp DR, Brandwein-Gensler MS, El-Naggar AK, et al. Carcinoma ex pleomorphic adenoma in World Health Organization classification of tumors, pathology and genetics, head and neck tumors pub. Lyon (France): IARC; 2005. p. 242–3.

31. Katabi N, Gomez D, Klimstra DS, et al. Prognostic factors of recurrence in salivary carcinoma ex pleomorphic adenoma, with emphasis on the carcinoma histologic subtype: a clinicopathologic study of 43 cases. Hum Pathol 2010;41(7):927–34.

32. Weiler C, Zengel P, van der Wal JE, et al. Carcinoma ex pleomorphic adenoma with special reference to the prognostic significance of histological progression: a clinicopathological investigation of 41 cases. Histopathology 2011;59(4):741–50.

33. Griffith CC, Thompson LD, Assaad A, et al. Salivary duct carcinoma and the concept of early carcinoma ex pleomorphic adenoma. Histopathology 2014; 65(6):854–60.

34. Rito M, Fonseca I. Carcinoma ex-pleomorphic adenoma of the salivary glands has a high risk of progression when the tumor invades more than 2.5 mm beyond the capsule of the residual pleomorphic adenoma. Virchows Arch 2016;468(3):297–303.

35. Hellquist H, Skálová A, Barnes L, et al. Cervical lymph Node Metastasis in High-Grade transformation of Head and Neck Adenoid Cystic Carcinoma: a Collective International review. Adv Ther 2016; 33(3):357–68.

36. Seethala RR. An update on grading of salivary gland carcinomas. Head Neck Pathol 2009;3:69–77.

37. Nagao T. "Dedifferentiation" and high-grade transformation in salivary gland carcinomas. Head Neck Pathol 2013;7:S37–47.

38. National Comprehensive Cancer Network Clinical Practice Guidelines in Oncology (NCCN guidelines). Head and Neck Cancers. Version 2.2013. Available at: https://www.nccn.org/professionals/physician_gls/f_guidelines.asp. Accessed April 14, 2016.

39. Byrd SA, Spector ME, Carey TE, et al. Predictors of recurrence and survival for head and neck mucoepidermoid carcinoma. Otolaryngol Head Neck Surg 2013;149(3):402–8.

40. Katabi N, Ghossein R, Ali S, et al. I. Prognostic features in mucoepidermoid carcinoma of major salivary glands with emphasis on tumour histologic grading. Histopathology 2014;65(6):793–804.

41. Liu S, Ow A, Ruan M, et al. Prognostic factors in primary salivary gland mucoepidermoid carcinoma: an analysis of 376 cases in an Eastern Chinese population. Int J Oral Maxillofac Surg 2014;43(6):667–73.

42. Nance MA, Seethala RR, Wang Y, et al. Treatment and survival outcomes based on histologic grading in patients with head and neck mucoepidermoid carcinoma. Cancer 2008;113(8):2082–9.

43. Brandwein MS, Ivanov K, Wallace DI, et al. Mucoepidermoid carcinoma: a clinicopathologic study of 80 patients with special reference to histological grading. Am J Surg Pathol 2001;25(7):835–45.

44. McHugh CH, Roberts DB, El-Naggar AK, et al. Prognostic factors in mucoepidermoid carcinoma of the salivary glands. Cancer 2012;118(16):3928–36.

45. Ali S, Sarhan M, Palmer FL, et al. Cause-specific mortality in patients with mucoepidermoid carcinoma of the major salivary glands. Ann Surg Oncol 2013;20(7):2396–404.

46. Chen MM, Roman SA, Sosa JA, et al. Histologic grade as prognostic indicator for mucoepidermoid carcinoma: a population-level analysis of 2400 patients. Head Neck 2014;36(2):158–63.

47. Schwarz S, Stiegler C, Müller M, et al. Salivary gland mucoepidermoid carcinoma is a clinically, morphologically and genetically heterogeneous entity: a clinicopathological study of 40 cases with emphasis on grading, histological variants and presence of the t(11;19) translocation. Histopathology 2011;58(4):557–70.

48. Hosokawa Y, Shirato H, Kagei K, et al. Role of radiotherapy for mucoepidermoid carcinoma of salivary gland. Oral Oncol 1999;35(1):105–11.

49. Ozawa H, Tomita T, Sakamoto K, et al. Mucoepidermoid carcinoma of the head and neck: clinical analysis of 43 patients. Jpn J Clin Oncol 2008;38(6):414–8.

50. Otsuka K, Imanishi Y, Tada Y, et al. Clinical outcomes and prognostic factors for salivary duct carcinoma: a multi-institutional analysis of 141 patients. Ann Surg Oncol 2016;23(6):2038–45.

51. Johnston ML, Huang SH, Waldron JN, et al. Salivary duct carcinoma: treatment, outcomes, and patterns of failure. Head Neck 2016;38(Suppl 1):E820–6.

52. Mifsud M, Sharma S, Leon M, et al. Salivary duct carcinoma of the parotid: outcomes with a contemporary multidisciplinary treatment approach. Otolaryngol Head Neck Surg 2016;154(6):1041–6.

53. Breinholt H, Elhakim MT, Godballe C, et al. Salivary duct carcinoma: a Danish national study. J Oral Pathol Med 2016;45(9):664–71.

54. Ko YH, Roh JH, Son YI, et al. Expression of mitotic checkpoint proteins BUB1B and MAD2L1 in salivary duct carcinomas. J Oral Pathol Med 2010;39(4):349–55.

55. Kim TH, Kim MS, Choi SH, et al. Postoperative radiotherapy in salivary ductal carcinoma: a single institution experience. Radiat Oncol J 2014;32(3):125–31.

56. Roh JL, Cho KJ, Kwon GY, et al. Prognostic values of pathologic findings and hypoxia markers in 21 patients with salivary duct carcinoma. J Surg Oncol 2008;97(7):596–600.

57. Shinoto M, Shioyama Y, Nakamura K, et al. Postoperative radiotherapy in patients with salivary duct carcinoma: clinical outcomes and prognostic factors. J Radiat Res 2013;54(5):925–30.

58. Jayaprakash V, Merzianu M, Warren GW, et al. Survival rates and prognostic factors for infiltrating salivary duct carcinoma: analysis of 228 cases from the Surveillance, Epidemiology, and End Results database. Head Neck 2014;36(5):694–701.

59. Martínez-Madrigal F, Pineda-Daboin K, Casiraghi O, et al. Salivary gland tumors of the mandible. Ann Diagn Pathol 2000;4(6):347–53.

60. Deng RX, Xu X, Zhang CP, et al. Primary intraosseous adenoid cystic carcinoma of the jaw: clinical and histopathologic analysis. J Oral Maxillofac Surg 2014;72(4):835.e1-10.

61. Zhou CX, Chen XM, Li TJ. Central mucoepidermoid carcinoma: a clinicopathologic and immunohistochemical study of 39 Chinese patients. Am J Surg Pathol 2012;36(1):18–26.

62. Li Y, Li LJ, Huang J, et al. Central malignant salivary gland tumors of the jaw: retrospective clinical analysis of 22 cases. J Oral Maxillofac Surg 2008;66(11):2247–53.

Margins for Benign Salivary Gland Neoplasms of the Head and Neck

Eric R. Carlson, DMD, MD[a],*, James Michael McCoy, DDS[b,c,d]

KEYWORDS

- Superficial parotidectomy • Partial superficial parotidectomy • Extracapsular dissection
- Facial nerve • Pseudocapsule • Linear margin • Anatomic barrier margin

KEY POINTS

- The superficial parotidectomy is the procedure for ablation of benign parotid tumors to which all other procedures are compared and vetted.
- The partial superficial parotidectomy and extracapsular dissection represent modifications of the superficial parotidectomy that are commonly performed in the management of benign parotid tumors.
- Unlike their counterparts in the parotid gland, benign tumors of the submandibular gland are most commonly surgically managed by removal of the entire gland and the tumor en bloc.
- Benign neoplasms of minor salivary gland origin are able to be managed with margins of the pseudocapsule of the tumor as well as the etiologic salivary gland tissue.
- The evaluation of a surgical margin, whether by a frozen section or by routine light microscopy, is always a collaborative effort between the operating surgeon and the surgical pathologist.

INTRODUCTION

Evaluation of patients with a salivary gland swelling should be quickly followed by the development of a differential diagnosis that must include neoplastic and non-neoplastic entities. The primary objective in the initial evaluation of a patient with a parotid swelling, for example, is to initiate the process of distinguishing a parotitis from a parotid tumor. When correctly performed, this approach leads to proper diagnosis and treatment.[1,2] This exercise is particularly important in the case of a possible malignant tumor of the parotid gland. As a whole, salivary gland tumors are rare compared with the overall incidence of head and neck tumors, varying internationally from about 0.4 to 13.5 cases per 100,000 people in the population.[3] Further, parotid tumors only represent approximately 0.6% of all tumors in the human body.[4] The parotid gland is the most common site of occurrence of salivary gland tumors, generally 60% to 75% of all salivary gland tumors in large series.[5–8] In an evaluation of 140 parotidectomy specimens, 102 (73%) demonstrated neoplastic disease and 38 (27%) specimens demonstrated non-neoplastic entities.[9] The investigators also examined 110 submandibular gland excisions, 17 (15%) of which were performed

Disclosure: Dr E.R. Carlson receives book royalties from Wiley Blackwell.
[a] Department of Oral and Maxillofacial Surgery, University of Tennessee Medical Center, University of Tennessee Cancer Institute, 1930 Alcoa Highway, Suite 335, Knoxville, TN 37920, USA; [b] Department of Oral and Maxillofacial Surgery, University of Tennessee Medical Center, 1924 Alcoa Highway, Knoxville, TN 37920, USA; [c] Department of Pathology, University of Tennessee Medical Center, 1924 Alcoa Highway, Knoxville, TN 37920, USA; [d] Department of Radiology, University of Tennessee Medical Center, 1924 Alcoa Highway, Knoxville, TN 37920, USA
* Corresponding author.
E-mail address: ecarlson@mc.utmck.edu

Oral Maxillofacial Surg Clin N Am 29 (2017) 325–340
http://dx.doi.org/10.1016/j.coms.2017.03.009

for neoplastic disease and 93 (85%) were performed for non-neoplastic disease. Therefore, when examining a patient with a parotid swelling, the likelihood of a neoplastic process should be highly considered. In contrast, examining a patient with a submandibular swelling is more likely to ultimately result in a diagnosis of inflammatory disease. Further, the cause of a sizable swelling of the minor salivary glands is almost always neoplastic. As many as 50% of these tumors are malignant, as typically occurs in the palate. An expedient investigation into the specific diagnosis of minor salivary gland tumors is, therefore, important to undertake.

The execution of surgery for all salivary gland tumors requires preoperative planning for the inclusion of a linear margin and surrounding anatomic barrier margins. Both types of margins are planned according to the specific salivary gland being addressed, as well as the specific surgical procedure being performed. In so doing, linear margins are quantitative and typically involve a calculated removal of normal salivary gland surrounding a tumor. Anatomic barrier margins are qualitative and typically involve careful dissection of the pseudocapsule surrounding the salivary gland tumor. Although the salivary gland literature commonly uses the nomenclature capsule, this article preferentially refers to this structure as a pseudocapsule because the host is responsible for the formation of this reactive tissue rather than the tumor itself. The performance of a superficial parotidectomy involves the inclusion of the anatomic barrier of the pseudocapsule without the intentional designation of a linear margin because the entire superficial lobe of the parotid gland is removed. By contrast, a partial superficial parotidectomy includes the anatomic barrier of the tumor's pseudocapsule, as well as a linear margin of normal parotid gland surrounding the tumor, for which dimensions are variably described in the literature. Finally, an extracapsular dissection (ECD) includes the pseudocapsule as an anatomic barrier margin but not a specific linear margin in this conservative removal of a parotid tumor. In all surgical procedures, at least a small area of the anatomic barrier of pseudocapsule of the tumor is likely to be exposed and is intentionally not violated during the ablative surgery.

Benign tumors of the submandibular gland are managed somewhat differently in that the tumor and the entire submandibular gland are excised with curative intent. As such, anatomic barrier margins are included with the tumor but no linear margin is planned because the entire gland is removed with the specimen. Benign minor salivary gland tumors are managed with surgical excision

of the tumor and its etiologic minor salivary glands, during which time the pseudocapsule of the tumor is likely to be identified and intentionally preserved. In addition, in the case of a benign minor salivary gland tumor of the palate, a linear margin of normal palatal mucosa is included at the periphery of the tumor specimen whose length is variably recommended in the international literature. Regardless of the specific benign major or minor salivary gland tumor, the inclusion of margins is executed in the best interests of a complete and curative tumor surgery.

This article reviews the particulars associated with margin inclusion and analysis in benign salivary gland tumor surgery. In so doing, evidence from the international literature, as well as anecdotal information, is drawn on as best practices to support recommended surgical procedures.

BENIGN PAROTID GLAND TUMORS

The international literature is a source of numerous monographs and observational reports of historical interest on tumors of the major salivary glands.[10–12] Early papers concentrated their comments on the details of histologic diagnosis and patient outcomes rather than on the specifics of surgical treatment and observation of margins. For example, McFarland[11] indicated in 1933 that treatment of parotid tumors centered on surgical excision although irradiation was becoming increasingly implemented. The publication of this paper preceded the widespread use of parotidectomy, as well as the establishment of specific nomenclature associated with this procedure or its required margins. McFarland[11] indicated that 30% of tumors recurred following excision. In his 1936 paper, McFarland[12] similarly used the term excision for surgical treatment of parotid tumors. This report reviewed 301 salivary gland tumors of which 278 were located in the parotid gland and 60 of these subjects developed recurrent disease following excision. Although it is unclear as to the specifics of surgical excision in these cases, it is possible that enucleation of the parotid tumors was performed because this procedure was commonly performed during that time. The 1953 report of Foote and Frazell[10] provided a review of 877 major salivary gland tumors, including 766 parotid tumors accumulated during the 20-year period ending in 1949. The primary emphasis of the report was to review the histologic classification and analysis of the natural history of a variety of tumor types that were primarily managed by surgery. As in the McFarland[11,12] papers, there were no comments about the type of surgery performed for these subjects. In 1941, Bailey[13] provided an historical review of parotid surgery, the shortcomings of enucleation of parotid tumors, the surgical anatomy of the parotid region, and the technique of total parotidectomy. Five descriptive cases were included in the paper, including 4 cases of total parotidectomy and 1 case of a facial nerve-sparing superficial parotidectomy. In 1958, Beahrs and Adson[14] reported on the surgical anatomy and technique of parotidectomy. Specifically, these investigators indicated that gradual knowledge of the biologic behavior of parotid tumors had been realized, including the results of inadequate operative procedures. This treatise provided a detailed description of the surgical anatomy of the parotidectomy, including the particulars of the facial nerve's course. Thereafter, Woods and colleagues[15] performed a study to compare the results of surgical treatment of 1360 parotid tumors during 2 consecutive 15-year periods, including 1940 through 1954 when local excision (enucleation) was performed and 1955 through 1969 when superficial and total parotidectomy were performed. There were 1132 benign tumors (83%) in the study. Sixty-five percent of the tumors in the period 1940 through 1954 were treated by local excision or biopsy followed by radiation therapy. Although the investigators focused their comments primarily on the concerning recurrence of the malignant tumors treated with local excision rather than parotidectomy, they also stated that superficial or total parotidectomy is best used primarily for benign tumors. All of this information ushered in the ability for surgeons to provide curative treatment of parotid tumors, simultaneously preserving patient form and function with a precise dissection of local anatomy. Subsequent investigators have modified the surgical techniques of the aforementioned investigators with inherent changes in the observation of linear and anatomic barrier margins as part of surgery for parotid neoplasms.

Superficial Parotidectomy

The time-honored superficial parotidectomy is the standard operation for the removal of a benign or malignant tumor of the superficial lobe of the parotid gland (**Fig. 1**). As part of this surgery, the entire superficial lobe of the parotid gland is removed with the tumor while intentionally dissecting and preserving the full course of the facial nerve, unless it is directly invaded by the tumor. The approach to the superficial parotidectomy is typically with the modified Blair incision of the preauricular and upper neck skin (see **Fig. 1**F). The skin flap is elevated in a plane superficial to the parotid capsule (see **Fig. 1**G). The sternocleidomastoid muscle is

identified and the posterior edge of the parotid gland is separated from this muscle. Inferiorly, the platysma muscle is divided and superior dissection is performed toward the tail of the parotid gland. Superiorly, the posterior edge of the parotid gland is sharply separated from the auricular cartilage. This sharp dissection is continued until the pointer cartilage is identified. Although the pointer cartilage does point to the main trunk of the facial nerve, the nerve is located more deeply in this region. A nerve stimulator is used at this time to initiate the process of identifying the main trunk of the facial nerve. The posterior belly of the digastric muscle is identified inferiorly and blunt dissection is performed in a superior direction to identify the junction of the posterior belly of the digastric muscle and the sternocleidomastoid muscle. The main trunk of the facial nerve is predictably located approximately 4 mm superior to this junction and at the same depth as this junction (see **Fig. 1**H). Once the main trunk is identified, careful dissection is performed superficial to this nerve and the bifurcation of the temporofacial and cervicofacial trunks is noted. Continued dissection of the deep surface of the superficial lobe and pseudocapsule of the parotid tumor is performed while exposing the entire course of the facial nerve and removing the entire superficial lobe of the parotid gland. The specimen is thereafter delivered (see **Fig. 1**I) and should be inspected for the intact nature of the pseudocapsule without tumor spillage, particularly on the deep aspect of the specimen adjacent to the preserved facial nerve (see **Fig. 1**J). The resultant tissue bed is evaluated for hemostasis (see **Fig. 1**L).

The superficial parotidectomy specimen includes as a margin the entire superficial lobe of the parotid gland containing the tumor and its pseudocapsule, with a resultant full dissection and intentional preservation of the facial nerve. As such, close margins are occasionally encountered and are frankly anticipated in the region of the tumor pseudocapsule adjacent to the preserved main trunk of the facial nerve and its branches, or adjacent to the parotid gland parenchyma sacrificed at the periphery of the tumor pseudocapsule. The status of these close margins has been studied extensively, particularly with regard to recurrence of the parotid tumor. Ghosh and colleagues[16] have assessed risk factors for recurrence of marginally excised parotid pleomorphic adenomas. They reviewed 394 subjects who underwent parotidectomy between 1980 and 1995, of whom 274 subjects had a diagnosis of pleomorphic adenoma. Of these subjects with a pleomorphic adenoma, 160 subjects had an adequate cuff of tissue (several millimeters) surrounding the tumor, whereas 114 subjects were

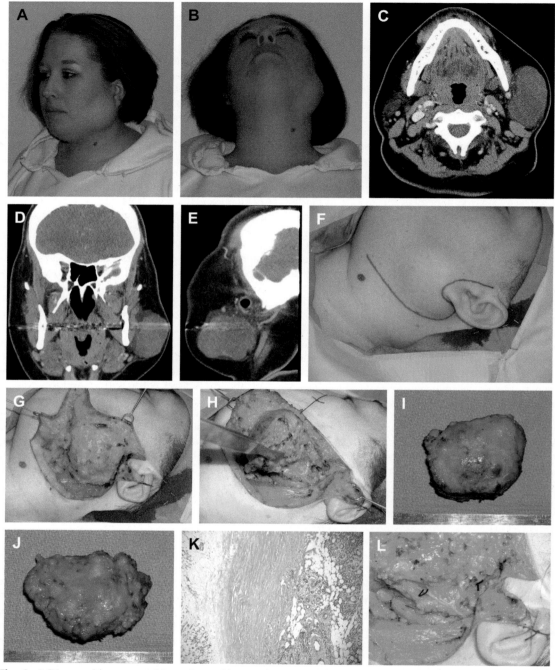

Fig. 1. A 34-year-old woman with an 8-year history of a slowly enlarging mass of the left parotid region (*A, B*). Computed tomograms were obtained that identified a homogenous mass associated with nearly the entire superficial lobe of the left parotid gland (*C–E*). The tumor is noted to exist superficial to the common facial vein (*C*), thereby permitting surgical removal of only the superficial lobe of the left parotid gland. Pleomorphic adenoma was suspected preoperatively due to the chronicity of the mass and its radiographic character. The patient was prepared for left superficial parotidectomy via a modified Blair incision (*F*). A skin flap was developed superficial to the left parotid gland, thereby exposing the entirety of the superficial aspect of the specimen (*G*). The facial nerve was identified approximately 4 mm superior to the junction of the posterior belly of the digastric muscle and the sternocleidomastoid muscle (*H*). A complete dissection of the facial nerve and all of its branches was accomplished that permitted delivery of the specimen (*I*). There was no tumor spillage encountered during the tumor surgery although significant pseudocapsular exposure was noted on the medial aspect of the specimen adjacent to the dissected and preserved facial nerve (*J*). Microscopic evaluation of the tumor specimen confirmed the presence of a pleomorphic adenoma with the identification of a relatively thick pseudocapsule that contained the tumor (*K*) (hematoxylin-eosin, original magnification ×100). The resultant defect from the superficial parotidectomy procedure is noted (*L*). Branches of the facial vein were carefully ligated so as to avoid trauma to the facial nerve.

considered to have a minimal marginal clearance around their tumors and were, therefore, thought to be at risk for recurrence. Eighty-three of the 114 subjects were included in the study because complete records were available for retrospective study. The overall recurrence rate in these subjects was 6.0% (5 subjects). Of the 5 recurrences, 3 tumors were noted to be widely present at the excision margin, 1 tumor was widely present within 1 mm of a margin, and 1 tumor showed a margin greater than 1 mm. This latter case experienced tumor spillage at the time of surgery. The investigators compared the cases in which tumor was widely present at the excision margin to those cases in which tumor was present within 1 mm of the excision margin. The recurrence rate was 17.6% in the former group and 1.8% in the latter group. In 33 of the 83 cases (39.8%), the surgeon considered that the tumor was adherent to 1 or more branches of the main trunk of the facial nerve. In 91% of these cases, it was possible, by careful dissection, to avoid having tumor present at the excision margin. The investigators concluded that the adequacy of excision of pleomorphic adenomas depends primarily on the presence or absence of tumor cells at the surgical excision margin. The microscopic presence of any thickness of pseudocapsule containing the tumor translates to a low risk of recurrence. In other words, the absence of tumor spillage during parotid tumor surgery likely translates to an effective and curative surgery. Therefore, they recommended that the surgical approach for pleomorphic salivary adenomas should be guided by the need to preserve vital structures rather than by an attempt to remove a cuff of normal tissue with the tumor.

McGurk and colleagues[17] similarly examined the clinical significance of the tumor pseudocapsule in the treatment of parotid pleomorphic adenomas by superficial parotidectomy performed in 95 subjects. The incidence of 2% recurrence led to their conclusion that careful dissection in close proximity to a pleomorphic adenoma need not lead to a high incidence of recurrence and that microinvasion of the pseudocapsule by tumor buds has limited clinical significance in so far as possible recurrence is concerned. Moreover, the investigators concluded that this surgical procedure embodies the principle of ECD in terms of management of the pseudocapsule in proximity to the facial nerve because the facial nerve is in contact with the tumor pseudocapsule in about half of subjects undergoing superficial parotidectomy.

The issue of the parotid pseudocapsular form has been extensively examined as it relates to vulnerability of the pseudocapsule at the time of superficial parotidectomy. This anatomic vulnerability specifically relates to the possible absence of a pseudocapsule, microinvasion of the pseudocapsule by the tumor, the presence of tumor buds, pseudocapsular lamellation, and bosselation. The latter is defined as a smooth bulging prominence at the tumor margin. Webb and Eveson[18] retrospectively examined 126 primary pleomorphic adenomas, of which 106 were located in the parotid gland. These investigators identified an increased pseudocapsular thickness in the presence of a hypercellular tumor compared with focal pseudocapsular absence seen in hypocellular tumors (69% of cases). In addition, they found that small tumors tended to be hypercellular whereas larger tumors (>25 mm) were hypocellular with an inherently thinner pseudocapsule. The investigators found microinvasion of the pseudocapsule with tumor buds in 11.9% of cases. All buds were bounded by a thin fibrous pseudocapsule and were closely connected to the main tumor mass. Bosselation was noted in 76 of 126 tumors (60.3%). Exposure of the pseudocapsule was evident in 81% of the cases operated in this series. The investigators concluded that salivary gland surgeons should be prepared for very precise dissection of the pseudocapsule to avoid rupture, particularly in the region of the facial nerve. Their findings indicated a frequently flimsy, variable, and uncertain border between a pleomorphic adenoma and the host tissue. They indicated that the superficial parotidectomy should guarantee at least some adequate tissue margin around the tumor.

Zbaren and Stauffer[19] evaluated the histologic features of the pseudocapsule of 218 pleomorphic adenomas of the parotid gland. Twenty-nine deep lobe tumors had been treated by total parotidectomy and 189 superficial lobe tumors had been treated by superficial parotidectomy. In 160 of these 218 cases (73%), 1 or more capsular characteristics, such as incomplete capsule (33%), capsular penetration by the tumor (26%), pseudopodia (40%), and satellite nodules (13%), were noted histologically. Moreover, the investigators categorized the capsular characteristics as a function of size of the tumor, including those tumors that were smaller than 2 cm (n = 95), between 2 and 4 cm (n = 110), and larger than 4 cm (n = 13). The observation of an incomplete capsule became more common with increasing tumor size. Capsular penetration, pseudopodia, and satellite nodules were most common in those tumors between 2 and 4 cm in size. Finally, the investigators observed focal capsular exposure in 80% of their cases. As such, these features should be anticipated when removing a parotid tumor and considered when determining the most appropriate procedure to perform to avoid tumor recurrence.

Almost all benign parotid tumors can be effectively managed with a superficial parotidectomy, but this procedure has been described as not being mandatory because higher rates of recurrence have not been identified in patients undergoing more conservative surgical procedures.[20] Although the enucleation procedure classically led to numerous recurrences, the ECD has been described as a minimal margin surgery with far fewer recurrences being described. At present, the partial superficial parotidectomy represents a practically acceptable compromise.

Partial Superficial Parotidectomy

When compared with the once performed enucleation procedure, the aforementioned superficial parotidectomy has demonstrated a dramatic decline in local recurrence of parotid tumors. Nonetheless, the superficial parotidectomy resulted in resection of a significant amount of normal parotid tissue, often leading to a loss of parotid function. In addition, temporary facial nerve paralysis due to complete facial nerve dissection was occasionally noted as part of the superficial parotidectomy. The observed complications of the superficial parotidectomy have led many surgeons to perform a limited or partial superficial parotidectomy. This surgical procedure removes the parotid tumor surrounded by a margin of variable dimension of normal parotid tissue while identifying and dissecting the facial nerve only in the vicinity of the sacrifice of the parotid tumor (Fig. 2). Like the superficial parotidectomy, the partial superficial parotidectomy may result in an ECD in the vicinity of the facial nerve dissection. O'Brien[21] retrospectively evaluated 363 partial superficial parotidectomies performed on 355 subjects with benign parotid disease. Tumors arose deep to the facial nerve in 40 subjects (11%), with 18 occupying the parapharyngeal space. The incidence of immediate postoperative facial nerve weakness was 27% (98 subjects), which proved to be temporary in 87 subjects and permanent in 11 subjects (3%). Some of the cases operated in this series were recurrent tumors with pre-existing facial nerve weakness. The incidence of permanent weakness of the facial nerve among the subjects with intact preoperative facial nerve function was 2.5%. Three subjects (0.8%) experienced recurrence of their tumors. The investigator indicated that partial superficial parotidectomy is the operation of choice for previously untreated localized parotid tumors lying superficial to the plane of the facial nerve because low morbidity was realized. It was pointed out that most malignant tumors of the superficial lobe of the parotid gland could also be removed by this technique.

Roh and colleagues[22] performed a randomized clinical trial comparing partial parotidectomy to superficial or total parotidectomy. They enrolled 101 subjects with benign tumors based on fine-needle aspiration biopsy (FNAB) and randomly assigned these subjects to 1 of 2 groups according to the extent of parotidectomy: 52 underwent limited partial parotidectomy (functional surgery group) and 49 subjects underwent superficial or total parotidectomy (conventional surgery group). The limited partial parotidectomy group underwent preservation of their greater auricular nerves and the main trunk of the facial nerve was identified. The overlying parotid tissue was dissected free of the nerve and maintained on the tumor with a linear margin of approximately 0.5 to 1.0 cm. The superficial or total parotidectomy group underwent a modified Blair approach to their tumor surgery and the greater auricular nerve was sacrificed during the surgery. A superficial or total parotidectomy was performed and all branches of the facial nerve were fully dissected. Twenty-one of 52 subjects (40%) in the limited partial parotidectomy group experienced early complications, whereas 49 of 49 (100%) subjects in the superficial or total parotidectomy group experienced early complications. Temporary facial nerve weakness was noted in 23 of the 101 subjects overall (22.8%), and was significantly more common in the superficial or total parotidectomy group. That no tumor recurrences were noted in both groups in a 4-year follow-up period, as well as other complications of less magnitude in the limited parotidectomy group, justifies this approach to benign parotid tumor removal. In addition, the partial superficial parotidectomy subjects realized favorable cosmetic, sensory, and salivary functions postoperatively, thereby providing additional justification for this modification of the conventional parotidectomy.

The recommended linear margin of normal parotid gland tissue included at the periphery of a benign parotid tumor is a subject of great variability when performing a partial superficial parotidectomy. For example, Plaza and colleagues[23] reviewed a case-control study comparing 25 subjects treated with partial superficial parotidectomy to 25 subjects treated with superficial parotidectomy, all of whom had benign tumors of the superficial lobe measuring less than 4 cm in size. The investigators specifically defined a linear margin of 1 to 2 cm of normal parotid gland tissue in the partial superficial parotidectomy subjects. Two cases of capsular rupture were noted in the partial superficial parotidectomy group and 2 cases in the superficial parotidectomy group. No recurrences were noted in either group of subjects with a

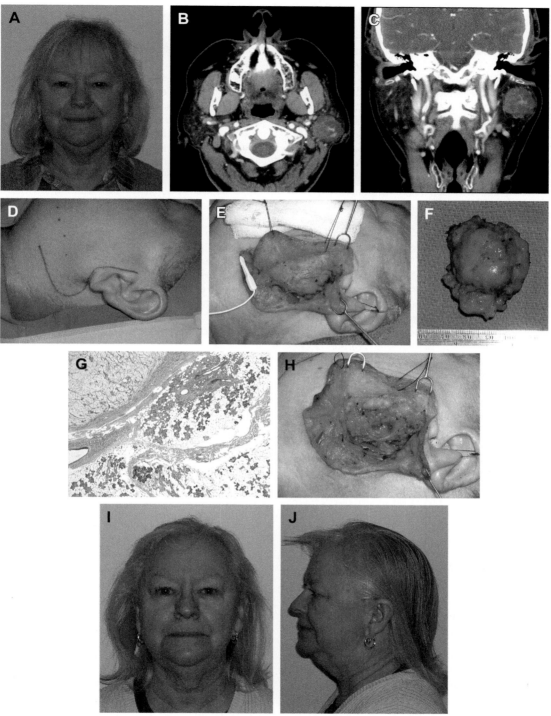

Fig. 2. A 63-year-old woman (*A*) with a 3.5 year history of a left posterior auricular mass. A fine-needle aspiration biopsy (FNAB) was performed that was not diagnostic. Computed tomograms were obtained that identified a 3 cm multinodular, heterogeneous mass located within the superficial lobe of the left parotid gland (*B, C*). With a presumed diagnosis of benign tumor of the left parotid gland, the patient underwent a partial superficial parotidectomy via a modified Blair incision (*D*). Removal of the tumor and 1 cm of surrounding parotid gland was accomplished (*E, F*). Microscopic evaluation of the tumor specimen resulted in a diagnosis of pleomorphic adenoma with a thin pseudocapsule surrounding the tumor and negative margins (*G*) (hematoxylin-eosin, original magnification ×40). As part of this surgery, the main trunk of the facial nerve was identified and dissected along with the surrounding parotid gland only in the region of the palpable tumor (*H*). The patient is noted at 2 years following surgery (*I, J*). No evidence of disease was detected and the facial nerve was intact.

minimum follow-up period of 4 years. Huang and colleagues[24] reviewed 320 total subjects undergoing removal of benign tumors of the parotid gland. Seventy-nine underwent partial superficial parotidectomy, whereas 241 subjects underwent superficial parotidectomy. These investigators observed a 0.5 to 1 cm cuff of normal parotid gland tissue while performing the partial superficial parotidectomy. No recurrences were noted in any subject in either group.

Domenick and Johnson[25] evaluated the proximity of the facial nerve to the capsule of 256 benign and malignant parotid tumors and assessed the diameter of the parotid tumor in predicting the proximity of the nerve to the capsule. One hundred and fifty benign parotid tumors made up this retrospective subject cohort that included 109 cases of pleomorphic adenoma and 41 cases of Warthin tumor. Of the pleomorphic adenomas, 53% were found to have a positive margin adjacent to the preserved facial nerve, whereas 37% of the Warthin tumors demonstrated a positive margin adjacent to the preserved facial nerve. For all tumor types, as size of the tumor increased the percentage of positive margins increased in a nearly linear fashion. A significant difference was noted between the diameter of the parotid tumor with a positive margin adjacent to the facial nerve and those with a negative margin adjacent to the facial nerve ($P<.001$). The mean diameter of a pleomorphic adenoma with a positive facial nerve margin was 3.02 cm, significantly larger than the 2.59 cm mean diameter of pleomorphic adenomas found to have a negative facial nerve margin ($P<.001$). Of pleomorphic adenomas greater than 5 cm in diameter, 81.82% had a positive facial nerve margin. The difference in diameter of Warthin tumors did not reach statistical significance ($P = .43$). Based on this information, the investigators indicated that the surgeon must be prepared to dissect the facial nerve from the capsule of many benign parotid neoplasms. Information regarding the presence or absence of recurrent disease in subjects whose tumors showed a positive margin in the pseudocapsule adjacent to the preserved facial nerve was not offered by the investigators of this paper. This notwithstanding, the investigators indicated that the results of their study showed no information to indicate that disease control was compromised by the presence of a positive pseudocapsule tumor margin.

Extracapsular Dissection

ECD represents the most conservative approach to parotid tumor surgery. A precise dissection immediately outside the tumor pseudocapsule is performed while intentionally not identifying and dissecting the main trunk or branches of the facial nerve (**Fig. 3**). This procedure has been referred to as a minimal margin surgery because only a small portion of the parotid gland is sacrificed with the tumor specimen. ECD should not be confused with enucleation that involves opening of the capsule with intracapsular removal of the tumor while leaving the capsule in place and not sacrificing any parotid tissue. Enucleation was abandoned due to high observed recurrence rates that led to the performance of the formal parotidectomy. As pointed out by Iro and Zenk[26] the debate continues as to whether ECD is justifiable as a less-invasive surgical technique. To answer this question, one must consider whether basic criteria are met: safe tumor resection with equivalent recurrence rates to other surgical techniques; lower or equivalent complication rates; safe, reliable resection in case of recurrence; and acceptable cosmetic results.

George and McGurk[27] have pointed out that 60% of parotid tumors have been estimated to lie on the facial nerve, such that an ECD of a parotid tumor is likely to occur as part of a superficial parotidectomy or partial superficial parotidectomy. In fact, Witt and Iacocca[28] determined that 21% of the capsule was exposed (range 4%–50%) in their review of 4 subjects undergoing superficial parotidectomy for pleomorphic adenoma. Their assessment of 8 subjects undergoing ECD for pleomorphic adenoma showed a mean of 80% capsular exposure (range 71%–99%). Because surgical protocol calls for preservation of the facial nerve, the result is frequently a dissection along the pseudocapsule of the tumor with no margin of normal parotid tissue in this region. It has become apparent among those surgeons commonly performing parotid surgery that recurrence is uncommon despite the close association of the facial nerve to the pseudocapsule of the parotid tumor. In their study of 156 consecutive subjects with benign parotid tumors who were operated with ECD, George and McGurk[27] noted that complications were rare, including permanent facial nerve palsy (1%), temporary facial nerve palsy (3%), sialocele (1%), and Frey syndrome (<1%). They reported that ECD is not suitable for malignant tumors, and FNAB was used routinely in the preoperative workup of their subjects.

In 2003 McGurk and colleagues[29] reported on 821 subjects with previously untreated epithelial parotid neoplasms in which the preoperative diagnosis and judgment for surgery was based only on clinical examination. The tumors were classified by clinical criteria into simple tumors (clinically benign) and complex tumors (clinically malignant).

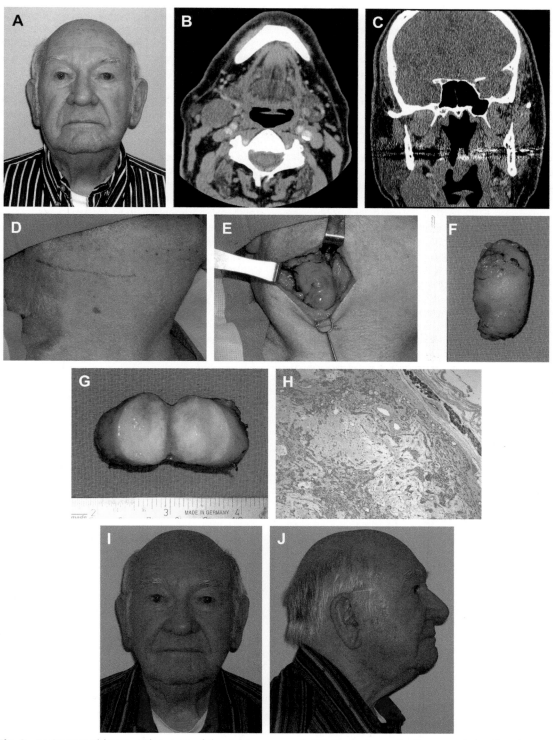

Fig. 3. An 83-year-old man with a mass of the right upper neck (*A*). Physical examination revealed a discrete mass that was indurated and associated with the tail of the right parotid gland. Computed tomography (CT) scans identified a homogenous mass (*B*) that was associated with the tail of the right parotid gland (*C*). The patient underwent ECD of the right parotid tail tumor through an upper neck incision (*D*) rather than a traditional modified Blair incision for parotid surgery. Precise ECD was performed to maintain the tumor's pseudocapsule, thereby avoiding tumor spillage (*E*). There was no dissection of the facial nerve during this tumor surgery. The specimen is noted to consist of a

Simple tumors were discrete, mobile, and measured less than 4 cm in diameter. Complex tumors were clinically defined as those greater than 4 cm, fixed to surrounding tissues, associated with facial nerve palsy, having deep lobe involvement, or those that were associated with cervical lymphadenopathy. Among those with simple tumors, 503 subjects underwent ECD and 159 subjects underwent superficial parotidectomy. Thirty-two of these 662 simple tumors (5%) proved to be carcinomas and two-thirds of these subjects had low-grade acinic cell carcinomas or low-grade mucoepidermoid carcinomas. Of these 32 subjects with malignant disease, 12 subjects had undergone ECD and 20 subjects had undergone superficial parotidectomy. The 5-year and 10-year cancer-specific survival rates were 100% and 98% for ECD and superficial parotidectomy, respectively. Of the 630 subjects with simple tumors and benign histologies, there were 10 recurrences at 15 years. Eight recurrences occurred after 491 ECDs (1.6%) and 2 recurrences occurred after 139 superficial parotidectomies (1.4%). The investigators concluded by stating that ECD represents an acceptable alternative surgical approach to superficial parotidectomy for most benign tumors due to no differences in recurrence rates and a reduced incidence in overall morbidity.

Barzan and Pin[30] performed a retrospective study of 349 subjects undergoing surgical management of benign parotid tumors with a minimum follow-up of 7 years. Two hundred and nineteen subjects had pleomorphic adenomas and 165 subjects had Warthin tumors. ECD was performed in 332 subjects and superficial parotidectomy was performed in 52 subjects. The total recurrence rate was 3.15%, including 7 subjects (2.3%) after ECD and 5 subjects (12%) after superficial parotidectomy. Cristofaro and colleagues[31] similarly compared ECD to superficial parotidectomy in subjects with parotid tumors. A total of 198 subjects were treated, 153 of whom underwent ECD and 45 of whom underwent superficial parotidectomy. Five recurrences (3.3%) were noted in the ECD group and 1 recurrence (2.2%) was noted in the superficial parotidectomy group. The superficial

parotidectomy group had an overall higher rate of complications, including facial nerve palsies.

Orabona and colleagues[32] retrospectively analyzed 232 subjects who underwent surgery for benign primary parotid tumors. ECD was performed in 176 cases and superficial parotidectomy was performed in 56 cases. The mean tumor size was 1.89 cm for subjects undergoing ECD and 3.49 cm for subjects undergoing superficial parotidectomy. Of pleomorphic adenoma cases, 103 were treated by ECD and 33 cases by superficial parotidectomy. Of Warthin tumor cases, 66 were treated by ECD and 22 by superficial parotidectomy. Capsular rupture (3.4%) and recurrence (4.5%) were significantly more frequent with ECD than in association with superficial parotidectomy (1.8% and 3.6%, respectively). Subjects undergoing ECD did not experience permanent facial nerve palsies or Frey syndrome. The investigators concluded by stating that ECD of benign parotid tumors is the treatment of choice for tumors located in the superficial lobe of the gland. This notwithstanding, the investigators recommended superficial parotidectomy for tumors larger than 3 cm and for recurrent tumors.

BENIGN SUBMANDIBULAR GLAND TUMORS

Tumors of the submandibular gland are rare, accounting for approximately 10% of all salivary gland tumors.[33] The first discussion of submandibular gland tumors in the international literature occurred in the 1936 McFarland[12] review of 301 tumors of the major salivary glands. This report reviewed 278 parotid tumors, 22 submandibular gland tumors, and 1 sublingual gland tumor. No specific comments were made regarding the surgical techniques associated with submandibular gland tumor removal. Because 50% of submandibular gland tumors are benign, a relative paucity of information exists on the surgery and outcomes of patients with these tumors. For example, Preuss and colleagues[34] retrospectively reviewed their 15-year experience with submandibular gland excision and noted that 207 subjects had non-neoplastic disease, whereas 51 subjects had neoplastic disease. Of the 51 subjects with neoplastic disease, 27 had a benign tumor and

---

pseudoencapsulated tumor with a small portion of the tail of the right parotid gland at its superior surface (*F*). The bivalved specimen (*G*) identifies signs consistent with pleomorphic adenoma that is confirmed on permanent histopathologic sections and demonstrating negative margins (*H*) (hematoxylin-eosin, original magnification ×4). Ideally, the specimen is inked by the pathologist before bivalving the specimen so as to avoid difficulty associated with margin assessments (see **Fig. 6**). The patient displayed acceptable signs of healing with maintenance of facial nerve function as noted at 1 year postoperatively (*I*, *J*). (*From* Carlson ER. Diagnosis and management of salivary lesions of the neck. Atlas Oral Maxillofac Surg Clin North Am 2015;23:53–55; with permission.)

24 had a malignant tumor. The investigators used a standard approach in their extirpation of these tumors that was not otherwise specified in terms of margins. In 1967, Eneroth and Hjertman[35] reviewed their experience with 187 cases of submandibular gland tumor between 1909 and 1965, with a primary focus on the 125 benign tumors in this series. Ninety-five subjects carried a diagnosis of mixed tumor. In 50 of these subjects, surgical excision of the tumor was performed, whereas 41 subjects underwent evacuation of the submandibular region (presumably removal of the gland and tumor) and 4 subjects underwent evacuation of the submandibular region and radical neck dissection.

Laskawi and colleagues[36] reviewed their series of 38 subjects treated for a benign tumor of the submandibular gland between 1966 and 1992. Thirty-five subjects were diagnosed with pleomorphic adenoma, 2 with lipomas, and 1 with hemangioma. Of the 35 cases of pleomorphic adenoma, 24 subjects were operated for primary tumors and 11 subjects were operated for recurrences. The 24 subjects operated for primary pleomorphic adenoma of the submandibular gland underwent total extirpation of the gland and tumor in 23 cases and 1 subject was treated with enucleation because the tumor was thought to represent a lymph node. Of the 11 subjects treated for recurrent disease, 4 subjects underwent total extirpation of the gland and recurrent tumor, and the remaining 7 subjects underwent removal of the recurrence because the gland had been previously removed. Thirty-one of the 38 subjects underwent proper follow-up examinations with the investigators that demonstrated no instances of recurrence. These 31 subjects included 21 of the 24 subjects operated for primary pleomorphic adenomas and 10 of the 11 subjects operated for recurrent pleomorphic adenomas. The investigators concluded that extirpation of the submandibular gland and its tumor is the therapy of choice for management of benign submandibular gland tumors. The linear margin in such a surgery does not require quantification because the entire submandibular gland is removed. The primary anatomic barrier margin is represented by the pseudocapsule of the benign tumor that requires careful dissection to avoid tumor spillage. As pointed out by Carlson and Lee,[33] preoperative imaging with computed tomography (CT) scans will precisely locate the submandibular gland tumor and guide the dissection of the pseudocapsule of the tumor. For example, tumors that are located within the submandibular gland merely require excision of the gland without concern for tumor spillage. The benign tumor that extends beyond the parenchyma of the gland must be surgically managed with a careful dissection of the tumor pseudocapsule to avoid tumor spillage.

In 2008, Roh and Park[37] proposed partial submandibular gland removal in their surgical removal of pleomorphic adenomas of this gland. They cited the trend in partial removal of the parotid gland for benign tumors to justify their suggestion for partial removal of the submandibular gland for benign neoplastic disease. The investigators prospectively studied 20 consecutive subjects with pleomorphic adenomas of the submandibular gland in which a 0.5 cm linear margin of uninvolved submandibular gland was sacrificed with the tumor. All subjects underwent CT scans and preoperative FNAB to document benign disease. Clear resection margins were identified microscopically and no cases of recurrence were identified in the follow-up period that ranged from 24 to 52 months with a mean of 36 months. The investigators concluded that this technique is safe and cosmetically favorable as prevention of a neck concavity occurs due to preservation of part of the gland. In the final analysis, complete extirpation of the gland with the tumor en bloc nonetheless seems to be the time-honored surgical procedure of choice for surgical treatment of benign submandibular gland tumors that represents curative treatment (**Fig. 4**).

BENIGN MINOR SALIVARY GLAND TUMORS

Minor salivary gland tumors are relatively uncommon neoplastic entities that represent the second most common category of salivary gland tumors in large series, with the parotid being the most common, followed by the minor salivary glands collectively. Next in prevalence are tumors of the submandibular gland followed by the very rare sublingual gland tumors.[6,38,39] Palatal minor salivary gland tumors are the most common anatomic site affected and most series identify a nearly equal distribution of benign and malignant tumors in this site.[40] An incisional biopsy of a palatal tumor is, therefore, required to plan proper surgical treatment that, in the case of a benign tumor, involves a bone-sparing, periosteal-sacrificing, wide excision incorporating 5 to 10 mm linear margins in the palatal mucosa and careful dissection of the tumor's pseudocapsule. In so doing, the periosteum and tumor pseudocapsule represent the anatomic barrier margins on the deep surface of the tumor. In most cases of benign palatal salivary gland surgery, the exposed bone surface is permitted to heal by tertiary intention. In long-standing cases of benign salivary gland tumors of the palate, the thin remaining palatal bone is sacrificed on the deep surface of the tumor specimen because retention of the thinned bone is often not technically possible or

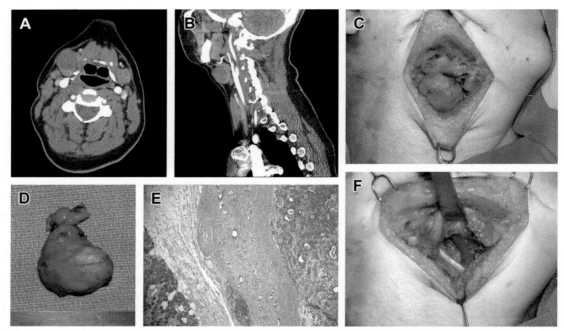

Fig. 4. The CT scans (*A, B*) of the neck in a 33-year-old woman with a 5-year history of a mass of the right neck. Near total replacement of the right submandibular gland by tumor was noted. Preoperative FNAB suggested the presence of benign disease. The patient underwent excision of the right submandibular gland and tumor en bloc (*C, D*) with careful dissection and inclusion of the tumor pseudocapsule. Pleomorphic adenoma was diagnosed histologically that was noted to be invading the pseudocapsule, although with negative margins (*E*) (hematoxylin-eosin, original magnification ×100). The defect is noted in (*F*).

anatomically meaningful. Immediate soft tissue reconstruction of the ablative defect is possible and desirable (**Fig. 5**). Benign minor salivary gland tumors of the upper lip and buccal mucosa are managed with a mucosal-sparing wide excision that sacrifices the etiologic minor salivary gland tissue with an intact pseudocapsule on the tumor.[40]

OPERATING SURGEON AND SURGICAL PATHOLOGIST INTERACTIONS: INTRAOPERATIVE CONSULTATIONS AND FROZEN SECTIONS

The management of salivary gland neoplasia requires that ablative surgeons personally interact with the surgical pathologist interpreting individual cases. This interaction serves the purpose of discussing the likely diagnosis of a preoperative FNAB and/or ultrasound-guided core needle biopsy of major salivary gland neoplasia. In addition, discussions involving preoperative incisional biopsy diagnoses of minor salivary gland tumors, intraoperative orientation of the tumor specimen, the utility of frozen sections, and the results of final pathologic tests are often undertaken.

FNAB of parotid and submandibular gland tumors has a time-honored role in the management

of these tumors. This technique is a reliable method of providing a preoperative classification of a benign or malignant salivary gland tumor, and is more sensitive and specific than preoperative imaging.[41] Christensen and colleagues[42] evaluated the results of preoperative FNAB of parotid gland lesions in 550 subjects, submandibular gland lesions in 240 subjects, and minor salivary gland lesions in 89 subjects. Overall, the sensitivity of FNAB in their series was 83% and the specificity was 99%.

To decrease the need for unnecessary surgery and to obviate a frozen-section biopsy, core needle biopsies of parotid tumors have become quite useful, especially in cases when the FNAB has not provided a definitive diagnosis. As with the FNAB, the core needle procedure can be accomplished as an outpatient procedure either with ultrasound or CT guidance. Currently, ultrasound is frequently the most reasonable technique because no radiation exposure is incurred by the patient. After years of trial and error, it seems that 18-gauge to 20-gauge biopsy needles, rather than those of a larger diameter, provide adequate tissue while producing fewer complications. Wan and colleagues[43] demonstrated a sensitivity of 98%, a specificity of 100%, and an accuracy of 98% in establishing specific tissue diagnoses by means of ultrasound-guided core needle

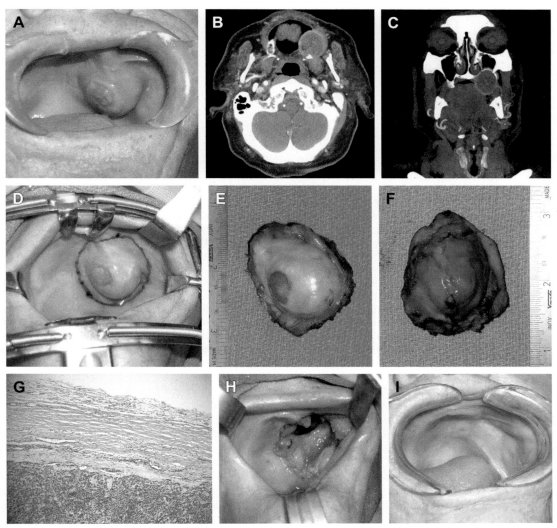

Fig. 5. A pleomorphic adenoma of the palate (*A*) in a 94-year-old man. The tumor had been present for at least 5 years according to the patient. Axial (*B*) and coronal (*C*) CT images identify a well-demarcated tumor that thins the palatal bone. A wide local excision was performed that includes the periosteum on the superior surface of the tumor (*D*). The planned mucosal margins measured approximately 5 to 10 mm. The specimen (*E*) identified an intact pseudocapsule on its superior surface (*F*). Permanent histopathologic sections confirmed the presence of pleomorphic adenoma that was noted to be invading the pseudocapsule yet with negative margins (*G*) (hematoxylin-eosin, original magnification ×100). Because the palatal bone was significantly thinned by the tumor, entrance into the sinus and nasal cavities occurred as part of this surgery (*H*). The left buccal fat pad was rotated into the defect based on the maxillary artery (*H*). The mucosalized fat flap is noted at 1 year postoperatively (*I*). Smaller benign palatal tumors customarily realize the preservation of the palatal bone.

biopsies of parotid lesions in a relatively large subject series. Complications incurred during this series were rare with no facial nerve damage, no needle tract tumor spread, and only 1 major hematoma identified. This article did describe the need for expert training in needle placement to spare damage to the facial nerve and tissue deep to the tumor itself.

Intraoperative orientation of a specimen similarly represents a crucial element of proper communication between the operating surgeon and the surgical pathologist. Such orientation will ensure that these individuals agree on the anatomic orientation of the specimen and on any areas of concern relative to the surgical specimen. In addition, the presence or absence of gross tumor spillage can be deliberated during the orientation session. Finally, the utility of obtaining frozen sections of the specimen can be discussed.

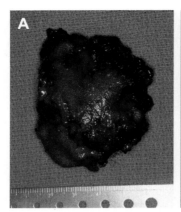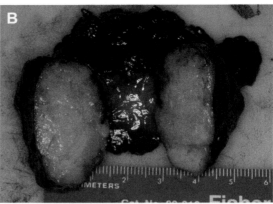

Fig. 6. The gross specimen (*A*) of a superficial parotidectomy for pleomorphic adenoma based on preoperative FNAB. As part of the intraoperative consultation process with the pathologist, the specimen was inked and bi-valved (*B*). The gross appearance is consistent with a pleomorphic adenoma and the tumor pseudocapsule is intact. The intraoperative consultation resulted in a frozen section being performed that showed pleomorphic adenoma that was confirmed on permanent sections.

The surgeon's request for frozen sections of a specimen is not a dogmatic exercise. Instead, it characterizes an informative discussion between the ablative surgeon and the surgical pathologist entering an operating room and, therefore, represents a second aspect of the intraoperative consultation process. Due to the relatively high false-negative rate of FNAB, many salivary gland surgeons will justifiably request frozen sections of their specimens. Olsen and colleagues[44] reviewed the results of 1339 consecutive parotid surgical procedures for 693 benign tumors, 268 malignant tumors, and 378 miscellaneous conditions at the Mayo Clinic between 2000 and 2009. Frozen sections were performed on every case and concordance of frozen section and permanent section diagnoses occurred in 1119 of the 1339 cases (84%). The investigators indicated that this cost-effective procedure is of greatest importance in distinguishing benign from malignant lesions because FNAB is rarely performed by these investigators. In some centers, the salivary gland specimen will be merely examined grossly and sectioned by the pathologist. These sections may permit the evaluation of the integrity and relative thickness of the tumor pseudocapsule, information that can be shared with the surgeon intraoperatively (**Fig. 6**). In their analysis of frozen sections of 721 parotid gland lesions, Badoual and colleagues[45] identified a specificity of 96% of 597 benign lesions. In fact, the benign tumors that were correctly diagnosed with high frequency on frozen sections included pleomorphic adenomas (95%) and Warthin tumor (92%), whereas the basal cell adenoma was correctly diagnosed in only 47% of cases. Finally, in terms of intraoperative decision-making, Mianroodi and colleagues[46] reviewed 85 parotid tumors

and noted that frozen sections resulted in an intraoperative change in surgical management in 6 cases, and 4 of those cases may have had more optimal surgery if frozen sections had been performed. The investigators, therefore, concluded their study by opining that the threshold for performing frozen sections in parotid tumor surgery should be very low.

The active role of the surgical pathologist in the operating room has become a well-established element of best practices in tumor surgery in the twenty-first century. The use of a frozen section is representative of the most definitive and currently available form of interaction between the ablative surgeon and surgical pathologist in an operating theater. In fact, this interaction should be part of all surgery and pathology training programs as part of best practices. Even though requests for the performance of frozen sections may not always be honored by the surgical pathologist, there is no doubt that such discussions are inherently collaborative.[47] Such discussions of relevance should easily be resolved by interactive communication. The pathologist must be aware of the various treatment algorithms available to the surgeon, just as the surgeon should understand the limitations of microscopic examinations of tumor specimens. Ultimately, both the surgeon and surgical pathologist should recognize that the frozen section represents a management tool rather than a diagnostic shortcut.

SUMMARY

Benign tumors of the major and minor salivary glands represent opportunities for curative ablative surgery and maintenance of patient form and function. The performance of a comprehensive preoperative workup with imaging studies and FNAB as indicated, the inclusion of the appropriate linear and anatomic barrier margins on the specimen, and the request for intraoperative pathologic consultation are multifactorial elements of benign salivary gland tumor surgery and represent a means to this end.

REFERENCES

1. Carlson ER. Diagnosis and management of salivary gland infections. Oral Maxillofac Surg Clin N Am 2009;21:293–312.
2. Carlson ER, Webb D. The diagnosis and management of parotid pathology. Oral Maxillofac Surg Clin N Am 2013;25:31–48.
3. Gregoire C. Salivary gland tumors: the parotid gland. In: Bagheri S, Bell B, Ali Kahn H, editors. Current therapy in oral and maxillofacial surgery. St Louis (MO): Saunders Elsevier; 2012. p. 450–60.
4. Witt RL. The significance of the margin in parotid surgery for pleomorphic adenoma. Laryngoscope 2002;112:2141–54.
5. Ellis GL, Auclair PL, Gnepp OR. Surgical pathology of the salivary glands. Philadelphia: WB Saunders; 1991.
6. Eveson JW, Cawson RA. Salivary gland tumours: a review of 2410 cases with particular reference to histological types, site, age and sex distribution. J Pathol 1985;146:51–8.
7. Spiro RH. Salivary neoplasms: overview of a 35-yer experience with 2,807 patients. Head Neck Surg 1986;8:177–84.
8. Ito FA, Ito K, Vargas PA, et al. Salivary gland tumors in a Brazilian population: a retrospective study of 496 cases. Int J Oral Maxillofac Surg 2005;34:533–6.
9. Gallia LJ, Johnson JT. The incidence of neoplastic versus inflammatory disease in major salivary gland masses diagnosed by surgery. Laryngoscope 1981; 91:512–6.
10. Foote FW, Frazell EL. Tumors of the major salivary glands. Cancer 1953;6:1065–133.
11. McFarland J. Tumors of the parotid region. Studies of one hundred and thirty-five cases. Surg Gynecol Obstet 1933;57:104–14.
12. McFarland J. Three hundred mixed tumors of the salivary glands, of which sixty-nine recurred. Surg Gynecol Obstet 1936;63:457–68.
13. Bailey H. The treatment of tumours of the parotid gland with special reference to total parotidectomy. Br J Surg 1941;28:337–46.
14. Beahrs OK, Adson MA. The surgical anatomy and technic of parotidectomy. Am J Surg 1958;95:885–96.
15. Woods JE, Chong GC, Beahrs OH. Experience with 1,360 primary parotid tumors. Am J Surg 1975;130: 460–2.
16. Ghosh S, Panarese A, Bull PD, et al. Marginally excised parotid pleomorphic salivary adenomas: risk factors for recurrence and management. A 12.5-year mean follow-up study of histologically marginal excisions. Clin Otolaryngol 2003;28:262–6.
17. McGurk M, Renehan A, Gleave EN, et al. Clinical significance of the tumour capsule in the treatment of parotid pleomorphic adenomas. Br J Surg 1996; 83:1747–9.
18. Webb AJ, Eveson JW. Pleomorphic adenomas of the major salivary glands: a study of the capsular form in relation to surgical management. Clin Otolaryngol 2001;26:134–42.
19. Zbaren P, Stauffer E. Pleomorphic adenoma of the parotid gland: histopathologic analysis of the capsular characteristics of 218 tumors. Head Neck 2007;29:751–7.
20. Zbaren P, Poorten VV, Witt RL, et al. Pleomorphic adenoma of the parotid: formal parotidectomy or limited surgery? Am J Surg 2013;205:109–18.
21. O'Brien CJ. Current management of benign parotid tumors – the role of limited superficial parotidectomy. Head Neck 2003;25:946–52.
22. Roh JL, Kim HS, Park CI. Randomized clinical trial comparing partial parotidectomy versus superficial or total parotidectomy. Br J Surg 2007;94:1081–7.
23. Plaza G, Amarillo E, Hernandez-Garcia E, et al. The role of partial parotidectomy for benign parotid tumors: a case-control study. Acta Otolaryngol 2015; 135:718–21.
24. Huang G, Guangqi Y, Wei X, et al. Superficial parotidectomy versus partial superficial parotidectomy in treating benign parotid tumors. Oncol Lett 2015;9: 887–90.
25. Domenick NA, Johnson JT. Parotid tumor size predicts proximity to the facial nerve. Laryngoscope 2011;1211:2366–70.
26. Iro H, Zenk J. Role of extracapsular dissection in surgical management of benign parotid tumors. JAMA Otolaryngol Head Neck Surg 2014;140:768–9.
27. George KS, McGurk M. Extracapsular dissection – minimal resection for benign parotid tumours. Br J Oral Maxillofac Surg 2011;49:451–4.
28. Witt RL, Iacocca M. Comparing capsule exposure using extracapsular dissection with partial superficial parotidectomy for pleomorphic adenoma. Am J Otolaryngol 2012;33:581–4.
29. McGurk M, Thomas BL, Renehan AG. Extracapsular dissection for clinically benign parotid lumps: reduced morbidity without oncological compromise. Br J Cancer 2003;89:1610–3.
30. Barzan L, Pin M. Extra-capsular dissection in benign parotid tumors. Oral Oncol 2012;48:977–9.
31. Cristofaro MG, Allegra E, Giudice, et al. Pleomorphic adenoma of the parotid: extracapsular dissection compared with superficial parotidectomy – a 10 year retrospective cohort study. Sci World J 2014.

Available at: http://dx.doi.org/10.1155/2014/564053. Accessed March 10, 2016.

32. Orabona GD, Bonavolonta P, Iaconetta G, et al. Surgical management of benign tumors of the parotid gland: extracapsular dissection versus superficial parotidectomy—our experience in 232 cases. J Oral Maxillofac Surg 2013;71:410–3.

33. Carlson ER, Lee AWC. Submandibular gland excision. In: Kademani D, Tiwana P, editors. Atlas of oral and maxillofacial surgery. St Louis (MO): Elsevier; 2015. p. 896–910. chapter 87.

34. Preuss SF, Klussmann JP, Wittekindt C, et al. Submandibular gland excision: 15 years of experience. J Oral Maxillofac Surg 2007;65:953–7.

35. Eneroth CM, Hjertman L. Benign tumours of the submandibular gland. Pract Otorhinolaryngol (Basel) 1967;29:166–81.

36. Laskawi R, Ellies M, Arglebe C, et al. Surgical management of benign tumors of the submandibular gland: a follow-up study. J Oral Maxillofac Surg 1995;53:506–8.

37. Roh JL, Park CI. Gland-preserving surgery for pleomorphic adenoma in the submandibular gland. Br J Surg 2008;95:1252–6.

38. Luksic I, Virag M, Manojlovic S, et al. Salivary gland tumours: 25 years of experience from a single institution in Croatia. J Craniomaxillofac Surg 2012;40:e75–81.

39. Wang X, Meng LJ, Hou T, et al. Tumours of the salivary glands in northeastern China: a retrospective study of 2508 patients. Br J Oral Maxillofac Surg 2015;53:132–7.

40. Carlson ER, Schimmele SR. The management of minor salivary gland tumors of the oral cavity. Atlas Oral Maxillofac Surg Clin North Am 1998;6:75–98.

41. Tryggvason G, Gailey MP, Hulstein SL. Accuracy of fine-needle aspiration and imaging in the preoperative workup of salivary gland mass lesions treated surgically. Laryngoscope 2013;123L:158–63.

42. Christensen RK, Bjorndal K, Godballe C, et al. Value of fine-needle aspiration biopsy of salivary gland lesions. Head Neck 2010;32:104–8.

43. Wan Y-L, Chan S-C, Chen Y-L, et al. Ultrasonography-guided core-needle biopsy of parotid gland masses. Am J Neuroradiol 2004;25:1608–12.

44. Olsen KD, Moore EJ, Lewis JE. Frozen section pathology for decision making in parotid surgery. JAMA Otolaryngol Head Neck Surg 2013;139:1275–8.

45. Badoual C, Rousseau A, Heudes D, et al. Evaluation of frozen section diagnosis in 721 parotid gland lesions. Histopathology 2006;49:538–58.

46. Mianroodi AAA, Sigston EA, Vallance NA. Frozen section for parotid surgery: should it become routine? ANZ J Surg 2006;76:736–9.

47. McCoy JM. Pathology of the oral and maxillofacial region: diagnostic and surgical considerations. In: Fonseca R, Marciani R, Turvey T, editors. Oral and maxillofacial surgery. 2nd edition. St Louis (MO): Elsevier; 2009. p. 213–7. chapter 23.

Margin Analysis
Cutaneous Malignancy of the Head and Neck

Donita Dyalram, DDS, MD[a,*], Steve Caldroney, DDS, MD[a],
Jonathon Heath, MD[b]

KEYWORDS

- Margin analysis • Cutaneous malignancy • Margins of skin cancers • Basal cell carcinoma
- Squamous cell carcinoma • Cutaneous melanoma

KEY POINTS

- Frozen section analysis of basal cell carcinoma and squamous cell carcinoma is best accessed by complete circumferential and peripheral and deep margin assessment (CCPDMA) or Mohs micrographic surgery. Pan cytokeratin stains can be used in challenging cases.
- Immunostaining with MART-1 has improved frozen section analysis of cutaneous melanoma.
- The use of immunostains has made significant strides in frozen section analysis of cutaneous malignant melanoma.

INTRODUCTION

This article focuses only on margin analysis of the cutaneous malignancy of the skin and discusses basal cell carcinoma (BCC), squamous cell carcinoma (SCC), and cutaneous malignant melanoma (CMM). The management of the neck and distant disease are beyond the scope of this article. It answers what is the appropriate surgical margin when excising these skin tumors, validity of frozen section analysis, and what to do if a positive resection margin is identified both intraoperatively and in the postoperative setting.

Skin cancer is a growing concern worldwide and has increased at epidemic rates as the baby boomer population ages. In the United States, it is the most common form of cancer, with 1 in 5 Americans developing skin cancer in their lifetime. Eighty percent of sun damage that will lead to skin cancer will have occurred before the age of 18 years.[1]

The 3 most common types of skin cancer are SCC, BCC, and CMM. Together, SCC and BCC are referred to as nonmelanoma skin cancer. It is difficult to accurately assess the number of new cases of skin cancer each year because they are inconsistently accounted for in tumor registries due to their high incidence and management in outpatient settings. The current estimate is that there are approximately 3.5 million cases diagnosed in the United States each year. More than $400 million dollars are spent in the United States annually to treat this disease.[1]

BASAL CELL CARCINOMA
Epidemiology

BCC is the most common skin malignancy and accounts for 75% of all skin cancers. This is a cancer

Disclosure Statement: The authors have nothing to disclose.
[a] Department of Oral Maxillofacial Surgery, University of Maryland, 650 West Baltimore Street, Suite 1218, Baltimore, MD 21201, USA; [b] Department of Pathology, University of Maryland School of Medicine, 22 South Greene Street, Baltimore, MD 21201, USA
* Corresponding author.
E-mail address: ddyalram@umaryland.edu

Oral Maxillofacial Surg Clin N Am 29 (2017) 341–353
http://dx.doi.org/10.1016/j.coms.2017.04.001
1042-3699/17/© 2017 Elsevier Inc. All rights reserved.

that develops in the epithelial keratinocytes of the basal layer of the skin. Despite being the most common, it has a low metastatic rate and accounts for less than 1% of deaths caused by cancer.

Areas closer to the equator have a high incidence of nonmelanoma cutaneous malignancy. The state of Hawaii has 4 times the annual incidence of BCC compared with mainland United States.[2] The eyelids, nose, ears, lips, and scalp are most susceptible to sun damage. It is clear that sun exposure plays a critical role in the pathogenesis of BCC. Race and ethnicity are also important risk factors. Light hair, blue eyes, freckles, fair complexion, Celtic ancestry (Scottish, Irish, Welsh), and Fitzpatrick skin types I and II patients have increased incidence of BCC.[3]

Pathogenesis

BCC is a neoplasm of hair follicles arising from keratinocyte stem cells, sebaceous glands, and interfollicular basal cells. Ultraviolet (UV) damage to the DNA creates mutation to genes, such as p53 for BCC and SCC, and the Patched (PTCH1) gene in BCC. Mutation to the p53 suppressor gene in these cells leads to inhibition of apoptosis and the development of skin cancer. This is seen is about 56% of BCC and alteration to the PTCH1 gene is seen in 30% to 40% of sporadic BCC. This gene has been involved in 2 inherited disorders: Gorlin syndrome and xeroderma pigmentosum.[4]

Preoperative and Risk Assessment

A patient with a suspicious BCC needs a diagnostic workup, which will include a history and physical, a complete skin examination, and a biopsy. The biopsy should include the deep reticular dermis. If the tumor is suspected to have extensive disease, then imaging studies are needed. Extensive disease is defined as tumor that involves bone, has perineural invasion (PNI), and has spread into the deep soft tissue. An MRI with

contrast is indicated if there is PNI. A computed tomography (CT) scan with contrast is indicated if there is bone involvement. The patient then undergoes a risk assessment to determine the preferred method of treatment.

A BCC is stratified as low risk if it is on the trunk or extremities. On the head and neck region, tumors on the forehead, cheeks, scalp, and neck are considered low risk. Primary tumors are those that are well-defined and have not been treated by other modalities. Additionally, there should be no evidence of PNI and histologic subtype should be nodular or superficial type.

The high-risk BCCs are those that are greater than 2 cm in the trunk and extremities, in the mask area of the face (around the eyes, nose, and lips), poorly defined, recurrent, has PNI, and shows an aggressive growth pattern (**Fig. 1**).

Management

Once a diagnosis of BCC is established, there are various therapeutic options available. In choosing the appropriate treatment option, size, location, histologic subtype, whether it has invaded local structures, and the presence of distant disease, will help to determine which modality is best. Curettage and electrodessication, cryosurgery, radiation therapy, Mohs surgery, laser surgery, surgical excision, photodynamic therapy, and medical treatment with interferon, imiquimod, 5-fluorouracil, and retinoids may play a role. However, to answer the question posed by this article, the focus is on surgical excision.

Surgical excision is the primary treatment modality. This is particularly true in locations where cosmesis is less an issue and where the tumor is well-demarcated.

The National Comprehensive Cancer Network (NCCN) recommends a 4 mm clinical margin for low-risk lesions.[5] For high-risk lesions, Mohs micrographic surgery or resections with complete margin assessment versus standard excision with wider

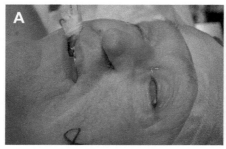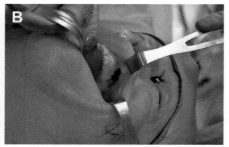

Fig. 1. (*A*) A recurrent BCC of the nose, which is considered high-risk because of its location in the mask area of the face. (*B*) The tumor has invaded into the maxilla. (*Courtesy of* Joshua E. Lubek, MD, DDS, Department of Oral and Maxillofacial Surgery, University of Maryland Medical Center.)

surgical margins. However, the NCCN guideline does not suggest a number for these wider margins.

Appropriate Surgical Margin

The appropriate surgical margin will eradicate all malignant cells in the clinical margin, as well as microscopic extension into normal-appearing skin. This would eventually lead to an optimal survival with low recurrence rate. To find the appropriate margin, normal-appearing skin must be excised.

In 1965, Gooding and colleagues[6] stated that BCC excised beyond 0.5 mm or 1 microscopic high power field had a recurrence rate of 1.2%. With a margin of less than 0.5 mm, the recurrence rate was 12%, whereas those with a positive margin had a recurrence rate of 33%. Another study looked at varying the surgical margin (1 mm, 2 mm, 3 mm, or 4 mm) to assess the rate at which each would yield a microscopic 0.5 mm clear margin.[7] After accounting for tissue shrinkage (approximately 24%), they found that an average of 4 mm will give an optimal microscopic margin in 96% of cases.

Wolf[8] sought the optimal surgical margin for BCCs by prospectively looking at 117 cases of untreated, well-demarcated BCCs. Increments of 2 mm were outlined on the normal-appearing skin surrounding the tumor. The tumors were excised using Mohs micrographic surgery. They found that a minimum margin of 4 mm was necessary to eliminate the tumor in more than 95% of the cases in BCC less than 2 cm. They did find that not all tumors required 4 mm excision in all directions. A 2 mm margin eradicated 70% of all tumors, with 3 mm eradicating all but 3% of tumors. They summarized that 4 mm will give a 95% confidence interval but it was at a cost of a significant amount of normal skin. They did not look at recurrence rate for these cases.[8]

A 4 mm surgical margin is not always feasible on the face, where function and cosmetic concerns are paramount. An analysis of 134 BCCs of less than 1 cm on the face was carried out by Kimyai-Asadi and colleagues[9] to address this question. An elliptical excision of 1 mm, 2 mm, or 3 mm was used around these tumors to achieve complete removal of tumor in a single excision. It was found that, overall, 20% had positive margins and needed re-excisions. At 1 mm, 16% had positive margins; at 2 mm, 24% had positive margins; and at 3 mm, 13% had positive margins. The conclusion was that for small, well-demarcated primary BCCs, a 4 mm surgical margin was appropriate.

Response to a Positive Margin

The positive margin has always been an issue of anxiety for surgeons because this is often discovered following surgical reconstruction of the defect. Negative margins may be impossible to achieve based on location of the tumor, pattern of growth, and depth of invasion. The question of how to discuss this with the patient can be a challenge: should it be observed or re-excised? Re-excision can be a major undertaking in cases in which the patient requires free flaps and/or local flaps to close the defect.

The incidence of recurrence following an incompletely resected BCC was found to be 41% in margin positive tumors. The mean time to recurrence was 24.6 months, suggesting re-excision of a positive margin tumor is prudent.[10] Dellon and colleagues[11] published a prospective study in which they noted that 93% of subjects with greater than 75% of their tumor cords containing irregularities at the peripheral margin had a 39-fold increase risk for recurrence. The risk of recurrence was also affected by the presence of a weak host inflammatory response (4 times risk), and ulceration (2.8-fold increase risk).

In a study that looked at 339 subjects with resection for BCC, 29 of which had a positive margin, none who had a re-excision within 2 months recurred, whereas those who did not have a re-excision all recurred.[12] These data strongly recommend the need for re-excision of those tumors found to have a positive margin.

Robinson and Fisher[13] reported on subjects over the course of 20 years who had positive margins following BCC resection. The investigators' found that the interval time to recurrence was 2 years. Superficial and keratotic lesion, 85% and 89%, respectively, developed recurrent symptoms within 2 years. It took longer for symptoms to present in men, those older than age 65 years, subjects with flap reconstruction, and those with aggressive BCC. This study did not stratify for low-risk BCC or location of the BCC.

A 2001 series reported no recurrence of low-risk BCC with positive margins over a 3.5 year follow-up (76% of lesions involved the head and neck).[14] On the other hand, Nagore and colleagues[15] found higher recurrence rate (26%) with positive margins than those with negative margins over a 5-year period (14%). A recent study in 2015, with a 70 month follow-up, reported a local recurrence rate of 26% in BCC subjects with positive margins (n = 6/25).[16]

SQUAMOUS CELL CARCINOMA
Epidemiology

SCC is the second most common form of cutaneous malignancy. It has an invasive nature and can metastasize to regional lymph nodes and distant organs. It occurs more in men and in regions near the equator, due to the cumulative sun exposure. Additional risk factors for SCC include chemicals (eg, arsenic and polycyclic hydrocarbons), human papilloma virus, scars, immunosuppression, and chronic ulceration. SCC occurs on body sites that have the most accumulation of UV radiation damage. It is seen more in men than women and usually in the 45 to 50 year age group. This skin cancer is not common among African, Asian, or Hispanics ethnicities; when occurring in these groups, SCC is not related to UV damage.[17]

Pathogenesis

SCC is a neoplasm of keratinocytes that constitute the epidermis and the epithelium of the adnexal structures. It can arise de novo within the skin or can be precipitated by UV damage, human papilloma infection, human immunodeficiency virus, immunosuppression, radiation, scarring, chronic ulcer, and exposure to carcinogens.

Preoperative and Risk Assessment

As in BCC, a patient with a suspicious lesion would undergo a similar preoperative assessment, including a history and physical, and a complete skin and regional lymph node examination. Imaging, such as an MRI or CT scan, is indicated. A biopsy is done to include the deep reticular layer. The lesion then undergoes a risk stratification to determine the modality of treatment.

There are some similarities with BCC when looking at risk factors for recurrence or metastasis. NCCN guidelines categorize SCC of the head and neck as less than 10 mm in size; well-defined; primary; without a history of immunosuppression, radiation, or neurologic symptoms; and exhibiting slow growth, such as low-risk tumors. Depth of invasion is critical, with superficial lesions classified as low-risk (less than 2 mm, Clarks I–III or histologic grades 1–2).[5]

High-risk SCC lesions include those greater than 10 mm in size, in the mask area of the face, poorly defined, recurrent, or in patients with a history of prior radiation or immunosuppression. Clarks level IV and V and depth of invasion greater than 2 mm both denote a high risk of recurrence (**Figs. 2–4**).

Management

For SCCs that invade into adipose tissue, surgical excision is recommended rather than curettage and electrodessication. The margin recommended for low-risk tumors is 4 to 6 mm. If there is a positive margin, Mohs micrographic surgery or surgical resection with complete circumferential and peripheral and deep margin assessment

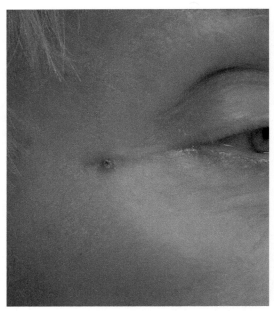

Fig. 2. SCC in the mask area of the face. The depth of invasion is 1.5 mm. (*Courtesy of* Joshua E. Lubek, MD, DDS, Department of Oral and Maxillofacial Surgery, University of Maryland Medical Center.)

(CCPDMA) is recommended. Mohs micrographic surgery or surgical resection with complete margin assessment is recommended as primary treatment of high-risk tumors. Radiation is reserved for nonsurgical candidates.[5]

Appropriate Surgical Margin

As in any tumor management, obtaining the appropriate clearance margin, which will confer long-term survival, is of utmost importance. Brodland and Zitelli[18] reported that a 4 mm margin was adequate for low-risk lesions. Cutaneous SCC lesions greater than 2 cm, histologic grade of 2 or

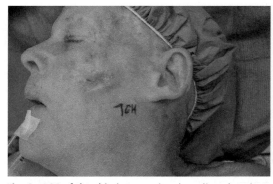

Fig. 3. SCC of the skin in a previously radiated patient. (*Courtesy of* Joshua E. Lubek, MD, DDS, Department of Oral and Maxillofacial Surgery, University of Maryland Medical Center.)

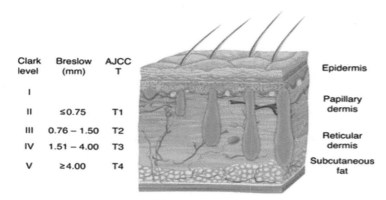

Clark level	Breslow (mm)	AJCC T
I		
II	≤0.75	T1
III	0.76 – 1.50	T2
IV	1.51 – 4.00	T3
V	≥4.00	T4

Fig. 4. Clark level, Breslow level, and American Joint Commission on Cancer (AJCC) T staging in relation to the layers of the dermis. (*From* Brunicardi FC, Andersen DK, Billar TR, et al. Scwartz principles of surgery. 9th edition. McGraw Hill; 2005; with permission.)

greater, invasion into the subcutaneous tissue, or a high risk should be excised with a 6 mm margin. The investigators make no mention of recurrence.

Tan and colleagues[19] reported on their incomplete excision rate in 517 SCCs and found that tumors excised with margins of between 2 to 5 mm had an incomplete excision rate of 6.4%, whereas those excised with 5 to 10 mm had no incomplete excisions. Although this study only had 26.8% head and neck SCCs, the ear and nose were the sites with the highest re-excision rates. Interestingly, most of the failures were in the lateral margin (62%) rather than the deep margin (3.4%).

In the United Kingdom, the practice has been to resect low-risk SCC with a 4 mm margin and high-risk SCC with 6 mm margin. In a large multicenter study, of 633 SCC using these margin distances, a 95% oncologic clearance was achieved.[20] Similar recommendations have been established by the French Society of Otolaryngology with the added caveat of increasing the margin to 10 mm if there are clinical risk factors for extension, such as incomplete primary resection, high histologic grade, extension into Clark level V, and PNI.[21]

The European Organization for Research and Treatment of Cancer (EORTC), European Dermatology Forum, and European Association of Dermato-Oncology published their consensus guidelines in 2015, which recommended 5 mm excision margins for low-risk tumors and a 10 mm margin for those tumors with a thickness of greater than 6 mm or high-risk features.[22]

Response to a Positive Margin

A positive margin is a difficult diagnosis both for the patient and for the surgeon.

This is especially true in difficult areas, such as around the eyes, nose, and ear. In an attempt to see which margin leads to most failure, 633 cutaneous SCCs were reviewed with 265 (42%) of these tumors being less than 2 cm.[20] Sixty percent

of these cutaneous SCCs were located in the head and neck, and a recurrence rate of 5.8% was reported. Of the 48 SCCs that were incompletely excised, 8% were positive at the radial margins, 68% were positive at the deep margin, and 24% were positive at both the radial and deep margins.[20]

Bovill and colleagues[23] retrospectively reviewed 676 SCCs. They found a 17.6% positive margin rate, with a positive margin being 1 mm or less. On review of the 84 tumors that were re-excised, 28.6% had residual tumor and the longer the time to re-excision (51 vs 72 days), the less residual tumor was seen. The deep margin was the most commonly positive margin, seen in 49% of cases. The tumor size, thickness, and location were the best predictors for residual tumor within re-excision specimens.

In a follow-up study, 79 of the 84 subjects were followed for a total of 27.7 months. Of those subjects, 21 had positive re-excision margins and 58 had a negative re-excision margin. Six of the 21 (29%) subjects who had positive re-excision margins had recurrence, whereas 3 of 58 (5%) subjects with negative re-excision had recurrence. In all, there was an 11% recurrence rate with 3 recurring locally and 6 regionally.[24]

FROZEN SECTION ANALYSIS FOR BASAL CELL CARCINOMA AND SQUAMOUS CELL CARCINOMA

Frozen section analysis has always been an important component of surgical management. Before reconstruction of a skin defect, whether it is with a free flap, local flap, skin grafts, or primary closure, it is paramount to ensure there is no residual tumor. Residual tumor cells under flaps can delay the visual recognition of recurrence. The question of how reliable is frozen section becomes a key factor in the management of these tumors.

Discrepancy between frozen section margins and permanent section margins can occur in 3 areas: sampling error by the surgeon taking the specimen, interpretation error by the pathologist, or specimen sampling error because only a fraction of a percent of the entire specimen can be evaluated on frozen section (**Figs. 5** and **6**).

A study comparing frozen sections with permanent sections for skin cancers, found that the results for negative frozen sections correlated with the permanent section result in 65% of cases.[25] Fifteen percent were negative on frozen section but positive on permanent sections. There were 8 cases (13%) that were read as negative on frozen section but tumor was found less than 1 mm on permanent section. In 4 cases (6.7%), no tumor was seen on both frozen and permanent sections. Overall, the accuracy of frozen section was found to be 85% in this study. Ghauri and colleagues[26] showed a concordance with frozen section and permanent section at 91.1%. However, both of these studies used conventional methods of sectioning the sample and did not give long-term follow-up data on their patients.

Further discrepancies found between frozen section and permanent section in high-risk tumors include those that are poorly differentiated, have PNI, and lymphovascular invasion.[27]

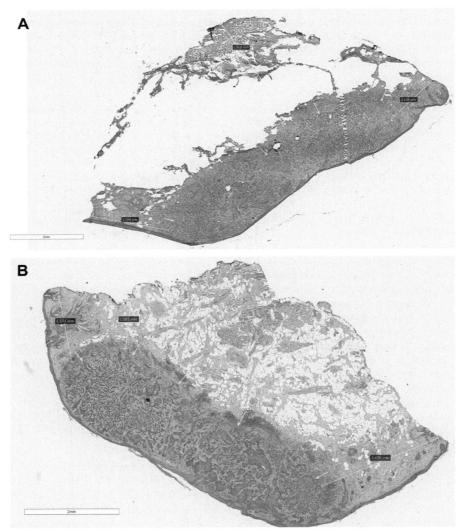

Fig. 5. (*A*) Frozen section of BCC (*arrows*) with negative margins (deep and lateral). Note the fragmentation artifact due to subcutaneous adipose tissue, which does not freeze at the same temperature as dermis and epidermis (hematoxylin-eosin [H&E], original magnification × 15). (*B*) The same section following formalin fixation and paraffin embedding. Adequate margins were obtained in this section (H&E, original magnification × 15).

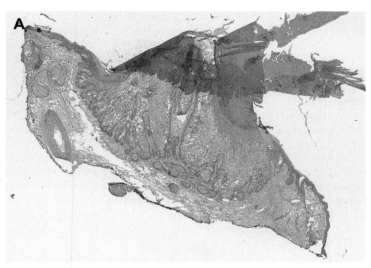

Fig. 6. (*A*) Frozen section of SCC (H&E, original magnification × 15). (*B*) The same SCC section in formalin and paraffin embedding (H&E, original magnification × 15).

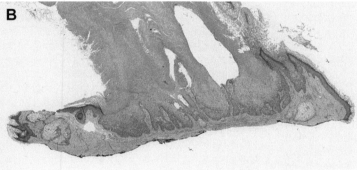

The method in which the frozen section specimens are taken by the surgeon also plays a role in accurately assessing a specimen. CCPDMA allows for all margins to be examined. This can be time-consuming and prohibitive in large tumors. Breadloafing technique (serial sectioning) only assesses those slices that are processed for frozen sectioning, with only a small proportion of those slices evaluated microscopically, using the typical 5 micron sectioning.

Overall, CCPDMA has been shown to be more accurate than the traditional, postoperative method of margin analysis.[28] Kimyai-Asadi and colleagues[29] found that the breadloafing technique (sectioning of the specimen at 4 mm increments) yields only 44% sensitivity in detecting residual tumor.

Casley and colleagues[30] looked at 150 cases of both BCC and SCC to answer this question. They found that the frozen sections were accurate to 97.7% when compared with permanent sections. They further demonstrated that assessment using CCPDMA had a better accuracy rate (99%) than

breadloafing technique (89%) in assessing margins.

The use of intraoperative frozen sections continues to be controversial. At times, it is considered optional because its reliability and effectiveness are debatable.

An Italian group looked at intraoperative frozen sections to see if it translated to improved outcomes.[31] Of 670 nonmelanoma skin cancers reviewed, only 71 had intraoperative frozen sections. The investigators found that, for these cases, 84.5% were completely excised, whereas the group with no intraoperative frozen sections had a success rate of 89.6%. The use of the frozen section was anatomic site specific (ie, eye and nose). The reason for such a high rate of false-negative could be attributed to the standard breadloafing method that was used for the frozen section.

There are situations in which Mohs micrographic surgery is not available or feasible and intraoperative frozen sections are the only analysis available before reconstruction can commence. In a retrospective review analyzing 1135 margins in 253 cases (cutaneous SCC and BCC) for skin excision using intraoperative frozen sections, compared with final review of the permanent sections, 58 (28.7%) of BCCs and 14 (27.5%) of SCCs, were found to be incompletely excised.[32] The investigators found that the lateral margin was more likely to be incompletely excised than the deep margin. After following these subjects for 2.9 years, there were 14 (20%) recurrences in the group with incomplete excision. Based on these data, this group has abandoned intraoperative frozen section by conventional technique.

Pan-cytokeratin antibody cocktails AE1/AE3, MNF116, and AE1/AE3+PCK26 have been used to further help in margin assessment in cases of BCC in addition to hematoxylin-eosin (H&E) stain. AE1/AE3 marker had the most consistent staining and was most helpful in complex cases and in areas of dense inflammation, which can obscure tumor cells.[33]

CUTANEOUS MALIGNANT MELANOMA
Epidemiology

Cutaneous melanoma is a malignant tumor of abnormally proliferating melanocytes. These cells from the neural crest produce the pigment melanin. Because of anatomic distributions and higher densities of melanocytes, melanoma usually originates in the skin and less frequently in the mucosa of other organs.[34]

Melanoma represents less than 5% of skin cancer; however, it results in the most mortality.[35] In 2016, the estimated new cases of melanoma were 76,830 with 10,130 related deaths, despite this region representing less than 10% of the total body surface area.[34,36,37]

Frequency of its occurrence is closely associated with the constitutive color of the skin and is the most rapidly increasing cancer in the white population. Worldwide, incidence depends on geographic zone, especially those areas with increased sun exposure. Most head and neck melanomas are seen in elderly persons and are rare before the age of 20 years. The median age is 55 years with a range of 40 to 70 years.[38] Up to 90% of head and neck melanoma occurs on the face and the incidence is 2 times greater in men than in women.[38–41]

Pathogenesis

The development of melanoma is multifactorial and seems to be related to factors such as fair complexion or sun sensitivity, excessive childhood sun exposure and blistering childhood sunburns, an increased number of common or atypical or dysplastic nevi (moles), a family history of melanoma, and the presence of a changing mole or evolving lesion on the skin.[42–45] The exact pathogenesis of cutaneous head and neck melanoma is still not fully elucidated, although long-term sun exposure to UV radiation seems to be the most significant risk factor. It likely involves a multistep process of progressive genetic mutations that alter cell proliferation, differentiation, and death, and that affect susceptibility to the carcinogenic effects of UV radiation.[46] Familial inheritance, potential tumor suppressor genes such as P16, and differences in DNA repair capacity contribute to carcinogenesis. In such circumstances, the damaged DNA activates the proto-oncogenes or inactivates the tumor suppressor genes.[47]

Preoperative and Risk Assessment

Cutaneous melanoma has been historically divided into both clinical and morphologic classifications. The 4 major histopathologic subtypes were developed according to the classifications discussed by Clark and colleagues[48,49] and later by Forman[50]. These subtypes include superficial spreading melanoma (SSM), nodular melanoma, lentigo maligna melanoma and acral lentiginous melanoma.

SSM is the most common morphologic subtype, accounting for 50% to 80% of cases, characterized by horizontal or radial growth. Nodular melanoma, the next most common type, shows an early onset of growth in a vertical direction and accounts for 20% to 30% of cases. Lentigo maligna melanoma is characterized by a prolonged radial growth phase and commonly occurs on sun-exposed surfaces with pre-existing large freckles (Hutchinson freckle). The tumor cells proliferate predominantly along the dermoepidermal junction and atypical melanocytes typically track down adnexal structures. Acral lentiginous melanomas are characteristically located on the palms or soles. Desmoplastic melanoma is thought to be an amelanotic variant seen with multiple spindle cells on histology and often lacks pigment. Although it accounts for only 1% of all melanomas, half arise in the head and neck.[50–52] Specific melanoma subtypes have not been found to be an independent predictor of survival.[53]

In terms of histologic classification, 2 systems have been used: the Clark and Breslow classifications. Clark grading involves a qualitative system to determine the depth of the primary melanoma based on the level of invasion of the dermis. In 1970, Breslow[54] identified tumor thickness, as measured from the granular layer of the epidermis to the deepest extent of tumor invasion, as an important predictor of recurrence and metastasis deemphasizing the Clark system. Tumor thickness is a measure that currently defines T staging. Because of this, an excisional biopsy is the preferred technique, especially for small easily accessible lesions to adequately evaluate tumor thickness.[52,53] A punch biopsy, incisional elliptical biopsy, or deep saucerization to the mid-dermis is recommended for larger lesions.[54] In recent years, Breslow thickness, mitotic rate, and ulceration have emerged as the most critical primary tumor characteristics, predicting outcome and guiding management decisions. It is these 3 characteristics that define T stage in the 7 th edition of American Joint Commission on Cancer (AJCC) guidelines.

As in other cutaneous malignancies, a complete skin assessment is warranted, as well as an assessment for melanoma risk factors. Currently, gene expression profiling is not routine outside of a clinical trial study. Therefore, in the absence of metastatic disease, *BRAF* testing is not needed for primary cutaneous melanoma.[5] Nodal assessment with radionuclide imaging, lymphoscintigraphy, or elective neck dissection is not discussed in this article but the reader should be aware of the risk of nodal spread in the face of cutaneous melanoma of the head and neck.

Management

The gold standard treatment of cutaneous head and neck melanoma is wide surgical excision with the goal of attaining negative surgical margins. Malignant cells may extend microns to several millimeters beyond clinically visible margins, necessitating a wider and deeper excision to ensure as complete a removal as possible. The American Academy of Dermatology also recommends that the depth of excision be carried out to the level of muscle fascia, if possible, or at least to deep adipose tissue, depending on anatomic location.[53] Various techniques to achieve complete histologic control include permanent section, frozen section, total peripheral margin control, and Mohs micrographic surgery.[54] For both in situ and invasive melanoma, permanent paraffin sections, rather than frozen section, have been considered the gold standard for histologic evaluation of surgical margins of melanocytic lesions.[55]

Appropriate Margin

Recommended surgical margins are based both on prospective randomized controlled trials (RCTs) and expert consensus opinion when no prospective data exist. Historically, Handley[56] described a 5 cm margin of excision, including subcutaneous tissue, fascia, and muscle. This was considered standard of care until the 1970s when Breslow and Macht[57] reported successful treatment in thin melanoma with a narrower margin of excision. Currently, there is a paucity of evidence, specifically for head and neck cutaneous melanoma. Furthermore, the evidence is extrapolated from RCTs for melanomas of other body sites. Of the 6 RCTs that have evaluated outcomes related to surgical margins of cutaneous melanoma, only 3 of these studies have included subjects with cutaneous melanoma of the head and neck.[58–65]

The Intergroup Melanoma Surgical Trial in 2001 examined the optimal surgical margins of excision for primary melanomas of intermediate thickness (1–4 mm) in a prospective multi-institutional trial. The 2 cohorts included either 468 subjects with melanoma on the trunk or proximal extremity randomized to a 2 cm or 4 cm excision and 272 subjects with melanomas on the head, neck, or distal extremities who received a 2 cm excision margin. A multivariate regression analysis showed that ulceration and head and neck sites were significant adverse independent factors. The trial concluded that a 2 cm margin of excision was safe.[59]

A large European multicenter phase III study addressed the question whether a limited surgery for primary malignant melanoma with a 2 cm margin was as good as a 5 cm margin. Nine European centers over a period of 5 years prospectively randomized 337 subjects with melanoma measuring less than 2.1 mm in thickness. There were only 16 lesions in the head and neck. The investigators concluded that for melanoma less than 2.1 mm thick, a margin of 2 cm is sufficient. A larger margin of 5 cm did not show a difference in local tumor recurrence rates, disease-free survival, or overall survival.[61]

Finally, the RCT by Gillgren and colleagues[62] included 9 European centers that evaluated subjects with melanoma thicker than 2 mm. Patients were randomized to resection margins of either 2 cm (n = 465) or 4 cm (n = 471). There were only 2 lesions in the head and neck. After a median follow-up of 6.7 years, it was determined that a 2 cm resection margin was sufficient and safe for melanoma thicker than 2 mm.

Based on these prospective RCTs, and review of available data, surgical margins in head and neck cutaneous melanoma have been established by the NCCN. However, outcomes associated with cutaneous head and neck melanoma are poorer when compared with all other body sites, with a higher rate of recurrence, shorter disease-free survival, and overall survival.[63]

Several studies have reported that melanomas located within the head and neck have a worse prognosis compared with melanomas at other sites.[64,65] In addition, melanomas of the head and neck are in close anatomic proximity to vital structures and recommended excision margins may compromise cosmesis, form, and function. The practicality of wide excision margins varies with the site of the lesion on the head and neck, and may not be feasible. For this reason, surgeons often rely on their own judgment when determining surgical margins in head and neck melanoma located on or near critical structures.[66]

The NCCN Clinical Practice Guidelines state that surgical margins may be modified to accommodate individual anatomic or functional considerations.[67] In a retrospective study by Rawlani and colleagues,[66] 79 cases of invasive head and neck melanoma were treated by wide local excision and followed prospectively for local recurrence. Forty-two patients were treated according to current practice guidelines and reduced margins (0.5 cm for lesions ≤1 mm thick, 0.5–1 cm for lesions 1.01–2.0 mm thick, and 1.0 cm for lesion >2 mm thick) were applied in 37 cases to preserve critical anatomic studies, such as the eyelid, nose, mouth, and auricle. The results showed that, in this small population of subjects from a single institution, local recurrence rates were comparable for reduced and recommended wide local excision margins.

A recent retrospective study of 108 subjects with thick (4 mm; T4), primary cutaneous melanoma of the head and neck demonstrated that wider margins did not significantly improve local regional control or melanoma specific survival.[67]

Future direction should include prospective studies specifically designed to study melanoma margins of the head and neck.

FROZEN SECTIONS ANALYSIS FOR CUTANEOUS MALIGNANT MELANOMA

Controversy currently exists as to the best way to evaluate melanoma histologically on frozen section analysis. Is frozen section with conventional H&E stain accurate or is there benefit to the addition of immunostaining?

In 1991, Zitelli and colleagues[68] looked at 221 specimens in 59 subjects comparing frozen sections and paraffin sections. They found a sensitivity of 100% with frozen section detecting melanoma and a specificity of 90%. Previous historical data have demonstrated similar results, concluding the accuracy of H&E stain on frozen section analysis.[69]

There are situations in which the use of standard stains can make it difficult to assess the margins. Patients with extremely sun-damaged skin can make it difficult to differentiate freezing artifact, actinic keratosis, and malignant melanoma. The use of melanocyte histochemical stains has helped to aid with this pathologic frozen section analysis.

Protein Melan-A, a melanoma antigen recognized by T cell 1 (MART-1), is an antigen found on surface of melanocytes. Antibodies against this antigen help recognize melanocyte differentiation. Human melanoma black 45 (HMB-45) is a monoclonal antibody that reacts against an antigen present in melanocytic tumors. Despite its high sensitivity, it can only detect about 40% to 70% of melanomas.[70]

Albertini and colleagues[71] reported on the sensitivity of these 2 stains for frozen section margin analysis. The investigators concluded that MART-1 was superior to HMB-45 when evaluating margins in malignant melanoma and melanoma in situ. A significant limitation to the application of these immunostains involves the significant time delay adding to operative costs (patient morbidity and economic), especially when procedures are performed under general anesthesia. MART-1

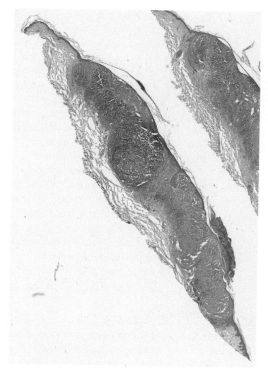

Fig. 7. Permanent section of a cutaneous melanoma of the face (H&E, original magnification × 15).

and HMB-45 staining can take more than an hour to complete. A 2005 study examined ultrarapid staining, which can be conducted in approximately 12 minutes, and found that that staining with MART-1 was more reliable than HMB-45 or S-100.[72] A 19-minute protocol for MART-1 stain showed similar results and reliability when compared with permanent sections.[73]

Etzkorn and colleagues[74] compared frozen section analysis with H& E stain, using standard techniques of either Mohs micrographic surgery, conventional breadloafing technique, or CCPDMA, in addition to the use of immunostain (MART-1). A total of 614 lesions were reviewed, of which 73% were melanomas in situ and 27% invasive melanoma. Using this technique of MART-1 immunostain, 34 (5.5%) of lesions were upstaged. The mean follow-up was 2.8 years with only 2 recurrences observed (**Fig. 7**).[74]

REFERENCES

1. Gardner KL, Rodney WM. Basal and squamous cell carcinomas. Prim Care 2000;27:447–58.
2. Stone JL, Reizer G, Scotto J. Incidence of non-melanoma skin cancer in Kauai during 1983. Hawaii Med J 1986;45:281–6.
3. Gloster HM, Brodland DG. The epidemiology of skin cancer. Dermatol Surg 1996;22:217–26.
4. Kim M, Park HJ, Baek S, et al. Mutations in the P53 and PTCH gene in basal cell carcinomas: UV mutations signatures and strand bias. J Dermatol Sci 2002;29:1–9.
5. Available at: www.nccn.org. Accessed December 12, 2016.
6. Gooding CA, White G, Yatsuhashi M. Significance of marginal extension in excised basal cell carcinoma. N Engl J Med 1965;273:923.
7. Thomas DJ, King AR, Peat BG. Excision Margins for non-melanotic skin cancer. Plast Reconstr Surg 2003;112:57–63.
8. Wolf DJ. Surgical margins for basal cell carcinoma. Arch Dermatol 1987;123:340–4.
9. Kimyai-Asadi A, Alam M, Goldberg LH, et al. Efficacy of narrow-margin excision of well-demarcated primary facial basal cell carcinomas. J Am Acad Dermatol 2005;53:464–8.
10. De Silva SP, Dellon AL. Recurrence rate of positive margin basal cell carcinoma: results of a five-year prospective study. J Surg Oncol 1985;28:72–4.
11. Dellon AL, DeSilva S, Connolly M, et al. Prediction of recurrence in incompletely excised basal cell carcinoma. Plast Reconstr Surg 1985;75:860–71.
12. Friedman HI, Williams T, Zamora S, et al. Recurrent basal cell carcinoma in margin-positive tumors. Ann Plast Surg 1997;38:232–5.
13. Robinson JK, Fisher S. Recurrent basal cell carcinoma after incomplete resection. Arch Dermatol 2000;136:1318–24.
14. Hallock GG, Lutz D. A prospective study of the accuracy of surgeon's diagnosis and significance of positive margins in non-melanoma skin cancers. Plast Reconstr Surg 2001;107:942–7.
15. Nagore E, Grau C, Molinero M, et al. Positive margins in basal cell carcinoma: relationship to clinical features and recurrence risk: a retrospective study of 248 patients. J Eur Acad Dermatol Venereol 2003;17:167–70.
16. Bozan A, Gode S, Kaya I, et al. Long-term follow-up of positive surgical margins in basal cell carcinoma of the face. Dermatol Surg 2015;41:761–7.
17. Gray DT, Suman VJ, Su WP. Trends in the population-based incidence of squamous cell carcinoma of the skin first diagnosed between 1973 through 1987. J Am Acad Dermatol 1990;23:413–21.
18. Brodland DG, Zitelli JA. Surgical margins for excision of primary cutaneous squamous cell carcinoma. J Am Acad Dermatol 1992;27:241–8.
19. Tan PY, Ek E, Su S, et al. Incomplete excision of squamous cell carcinoma of the skin: A prospective observational study. Plast Reconstr Surg 2007;120:910–6.
20. Khan AA, Potter M, Cubitt JJ, et al. Guidelines for excision of cutaneous scc cancers in the UK: the best cut is the deepest. J Plast Reconstr Aesthet Surg 2013;66:467–71.
21. Durbec M, Couloigner V, Tronche S, et al, SFORL Work Group. Guidelines of the French Society of Otorhinolaryngology (SFORL), short version. Extension assessment and principles of resection in cutaneous head and neck tumors. Eur Ann Otorhinolaryngol Head Neck Dis 2017;131:375–83.
22. Stratigos A, Garbe C, Lebbe C, et al. Diagnosis and treatment of invasive squamous cell carcinoma of the skin: European consensus-based interdisciplinary guideline. Eur J Cancer 2015;51:1989–2007.
23. Bovill ES, Cullen KW, Barrett W. Clinical and histological findings in re-excision of incompletely excised cutaneous squamous cell carcinoma. J Plast Reconstr Aesthet Surg 2009;62:457–61.
24. Bovill ES, Banwell PE. Re-excision of incompletely excised cutaneous squamous cell carcinoma: Histological findings influence prognosis. J Plast Reconstr Aesthet Surg 2012;65:1390–5.
25. Manstein ME, Manstein CH, Smith R. How accurate are frozen sections for skin cancers. Ann Plast Surg 2003;50:607–9.
26. Ghauri RR, Gunter AA, Weber RA. Frozen section analysis in the management of skin cancers. Ann Plast Surg 1999;43:156–60.
27. Chambers KJ, Kraft S, Emerick K. Evaluation of frozen sections margins in high risk squamous cell

carcinomas of the head and neck. Laryngoscope 2015;125:636–9.

28. Smith-Zagone MJ, Schwartz MR. Frozen section of skin specimens. Arch Pathol Lab Med 2005;129: 1536–43.

29. Kimyai-Asadi A, Goldberg LH, Ming HJ. Accuracy of serial transverse cross sections in detecting residual basal cell carcinoma at the surgical margins of an elliptical excision specimen. J Am Acad Dermatol 2005;53:469–74.

30. Casley AJ, Theile DR, Lambie D. The use of frozen section in the excision of Cutaneous Malignancy: A Queensland experience. Ann Plast Surg 2013;71: 386–9.

31. Nicoletti G, Brenta F, Malovini A, et al. Study to determine whether intra-operative frozen section biopsy improves surgical treatment of non-melanoma skin cancer. Mol Clinic Oncol 2013;1:390–4.

32. Moncrieff MD, Shah AK, Igali L, et al. False negative rate of intra-operative frozen section margin analysis for complete head and neck non melanoma skin cancer excision. Clin Exp Dermatol 2015;40:834–8.

33. Orchard GE, Wojcik K, Shams F. Pan-cytokeratin markers for rapid frozen section immunocytochemistry from head and facial Mohs cases of basal cell carcinoma: a comparison and evaluation to determine the marker of choice. Br J Biomed Sci 2015; 72:61–6.

34. Golger A, Young DS, Ghazarian D. Epidemiologic features and prognostic factors of cutaneous head and neck melanoma: a population–based study. Arch Otolaryngol Head Neck Surg 2007;133:442–7.

35. American Cancer Society. Cancer facts and figures 2014. Atlanta (GA): American Cancer Society; 2014. Available at: https://www.cancer.org/research/cancer-facts-statistics/all-cancer-facts-figures/cancer-facts-figures-2014.html. Accessed December 12, 2016.

36. American Cancer Society. Cancer facts and figures 2016. Atlanta (GA): American Cancer Society; 2016. Available at: https://www.cancer.org/content/dam/cancer-org/research/cancer-facts-and-statistics/annual-cancer-facts-and-figures/2016/cancer-facts-and-figures-2016.pdf. Accessed February 28, 2016.

37. Andtbacka RH, Agarwala SS, Olilla DW, et al. Cutaneous head and neck melanoma in OPTiM, a randomized phase 3 trial of talimogene laherparepvec versus granulocyte-macrophage-colony-stimulating factor for the treatment of unresected stage IIIB/IIIC/IV melanoma. Head Neck 2016; 38(12):1752–8. Published online 2016 in Wiley Online Library. Available at: wileyonlinelibrary.com. Accessed December 29, 2016.

38. Vikey AK, Vikey D. Primary malignant melanoma, of head and neck. A comprehensive review of literature. Oral Oncol 2012;48:399–403.

39. Hoersch B, Leiter U, Garbe C. Is head and neck melanoma a distinct entity? A clinical registry based comparative study in 5702 patients with melanoma. Br J Dermatol 2006;155:771–7.

40. Shashanka R, Smitha BR. Head and neck melanoma. ISRN Surg 2012;2012:948302.

41. Franklin JD, Reynolds VH, Bowers DG Jr. Cutaneous melanoma of the head and neck. Clin Plast Surg 1976;3:413–27.

42. Carlson GW, Murray DR, Lyles RH. Sentinel lymph node biopsy in the management of cutaneous head and neck melanoma. Plast Reconstr Surg 2005;115:721–8.

43. Sober AJ, Fitzpatrick TB, Mihm MC. Early recognition of cutaneous melanoma. JAMA 1979;242: 2795–9.

44. Rhodes AR, Weinstock MA, Fitzpatrick TB, et al. Risk factors for cutaneous melanoma. A practical method of recognizing predisposed individuals. JAMA 1987; 258:3146–54.

45. Williams ML, Sagebiel RW. Melanoma risk factors and atypical moles. West J Med 1994;160:343–50.

46. Demierre MF, Nathanson L. Chemoprevention of melanoma: an unexplored strategy. J Clin Oncol 2003;21:158–65.

47. Waldman V, Bock M, Jackel A, et al. Pathogenesis of malignant melanoma: molecular biology aspect. Hautarzt 1999;50:398–405.

48. Clark WH, From L, Bernadino EA, et al. The histogenesis and biologic behavior of primary malignant melanomas of the skin. Cancer Res 1969; 29:705–26.

49. Clark WH, Elder DE, Van Horn M. The biologic forms of malignant melanoma. Hum Pathol 1986;17:443–50.

50. Forman S, Ferringer T, Peckham S. Is superficial spreading melanoma still the most common form of malignant melanoma. J Am Acad Dermatol 2008;58:1013–20.

51. Au A, Ariyan S. Melanoma of the head and neck. J Craniofac Surg 2011;22:421–9.

52. Cheriyan J, Wernberg J, Urquhart A. Head and neck melanoma. Surg Clin North Am 2014;94:1091–113.

53. Zenga J, Nussenbaum B, Cornelius L, et al. Management controversies in head and neck melanoma. A systematic review. JAMA Facial Plast Surg 2017; 19(1):53–62. Published Online. jamafacial. Accessed December 20, 2016.

54. Breslow A. Thickness, cross-sectional areas and depth of invasion in the prognosis of cutaneous melanoma. Annals of Surgery 1970;172:902–8.

55. Prieto VG, Argenyi ZB, Barnhill RL, et al. Are en face frozen sections accurate for diagnosing margin status in melanocytic lesions? Am J Clin Pathol 2003; 120:203–8.

56. Handley WS. The pathology of melanocytic growths in relation to their operative treatment. Lecture II. Lancet 1907;1:996.

57. Breslow A, Macht SD. Optimal size of resection margin for thin cutaneous melanoma. Surg Gynecol Obstet 1977;145:691–2.

58. Cohn-Cedermark G, Rutqvist LE, Andersson R. Long term results of a randomized study by the Swedish Melanoma Study Group on 2-cm vs 5-cm resection margins for patients with cutaneous melanoma with a tumor thickness of 0.8-2.0 mm. Cancer 2000;89:1495–501.

59. Balch CM, Soong SJ, Smith T. Investigators from the intergroup melanoma surgical trial. Long-term results of a prospective surgical trial comparing 2 cm vs 4 cm excision margins for 740 patients with 1-4 mm melanomas. Ann Surg Oncol 2001;8:101–8.

60. Khayat D, Rixe O, Martin G, et al, French Group of Research on Malignant Melanoma. Surgical margins in cutaneous melanoma (2 cm vs 5 cm for lesions measuring less than 2.1-mm thick). Cancer 2003; 97:1941–6.

61. Thomas JM, Newton-Bishop J, A'Hern R, United Kingdom Melanoma Study Group, British Association of Plastic Surgeons, Scottish Cancer Therapy Network. Excision margins in high-risk malignant melanoma. N Engl J Med 2004;350:757–66.

62. Gillgren P, Drzewiecki KT, Niin M. 2-cm vs 4-cm surgical excision margins for primary cutaneous melanoma thicker than 2 mm: a randomised, multicentre trial. Lancet 2011;378:1635–42.

63. Fadaki N, Li R, Parrett B. Is head and neck melanoma different from trunk and extremity melanomas with respect to sentinel lymph node status and clinical outcome? Ann Surg Oncol 2013;20:3089–97.

64. Lachiewicz AM, Berwick M, Wiggins CL, et al. Survival differences between patients with scalp or neck melanoma and those with melanoma of other sites in the Surveillance, Epidemiology, and End Results (SEER) program. Arch Dermatol 2008;144: 515–21.

65. Tseng WH, Martinez SR. Tumor location predicts survival in cutaneous head and neck melanoma. J Surg Res 2011;167:192–8.

66. Rawlani R, Rawlani V, Qureshi H. Reducing margins of wide local excision in head and neck melanoma for function and cosmesis: 5 year local recurrence free survival. J Surg Oncol 2015;111:795–9.

67. National Comprehensive Cancer Network. Practice guidelines in oncology: melanoma. Available at: www.nccn.org. Accessed December 13, 2016.

68. Zitelli JA, Moy RL, Abell E. The reliability of frozen sections in the evaluation of surgical margins for melanoma. J Am Acad Dermatol 1991;24:102–6.

69. Little JH, Davis NC. Frozen section diagnosis of suspected malignant melanomas of the skin. Cancer 1974;34:1163–72.

70. Mahmood MN, Lee MW, Linden MD, et al. Diagnostic value of HMB-45 and anti-melan a staining of sentinel lymph nodes with isolated positive cells. Mod Pathol 2002;15:1288–93.

71. Albertini JG, Elston DM, Libow LF, et al. Mohs micrographic surgery for melanoma: a case series, a comparative study of immunostains, an informative case report and a unique mapping technique. Dermatol Surg 2002;28:656–65.

72. Davis DA, Kurtz KA, Robinson RA. Ultra-rapid staining for cutaneous melanoma: study and protocol. Dermatol Surg 2005;31:753–6.

73. Cherpelis BS, Moore R, Ladd S, et al. Comparison of MART-1 frozen sections to permanent sections using a rapid 19-Minute protocol. Dermatol Surg 2009;35: 207–13.

74. Etzkorn JR, Sobanko JF, Elenitsas R, et al. Low recurrence rates for in situ and invasive melanomas using Mohs micrographic surgery with melanoma antigen recognized by T cells 1 (MART-1) immunostaining: tissue processing methodology to optimize pathologic staging and margin assessment. J Am Acad Dermatol 2015;72:840–50.

Margin Analysis
Sarcoma of the Head and Neck

Raafat F. Makary, MBBCh (MD), PhD[a], Arun Gopinath, MD[b,*],
Michael R. Markiewicz, DDS, MPH, MD[c,d], Rui Fernandes, MD, DMD[e]

KEYWORDS

- Head and neck • Sarcoma • Histologic types • Resection margin • Prognosis

KEY POINTS

- Head and neck sarcomas are rare but are associated with significant morbidity/mortality and management difficulties.
- These tumors are best managed in a multidisciplinary setting.
- Open or core biopsy is essential for histologic diagnosis and grading. Based on histology, the tumors are divided into 3 categories; low grade, intermediate grade, and high grade, which helps in guiding therapy.
- Complete surgical tumor resection with negative margins at the first attempt is the best chance for potential cure.
- In most patients, except those with small resectable low-grade lesions, adjuvant radiotherapy and chemotherapy is added to maximize local control with variable results.

INTRODUCTION

Sarcomas are malignancies arising from mesenchymal (nonepithelial) tissue and are broadly classified into sarcomas of soft tissue and bone. Soft tissue sarcomas can arise from muscle, blood vessels, nerves, fat, and fibroconnective tissues. Sarcomas of bone are mainly osteosarcoma, chondrosarcomas (CS), and Ewing sarcoma (EWS).

Sarcomas are rare compared with carcinoma, accounting for 1% to 2% of all head and neck (HN) malignancies, of which approximately 80% originate from soft tissues and 20% from bone.[1]

Although rare in the HN, they represent an important but heterogeneous group of tumors that may be associated with management challenges and risk for morbidity/mortality.

HISTOLOGIC TYPES AND CLASSIFICATION OF HEAD AND NECK SARCOMAS

More than 60 histologic subtypes of bone and soft tissue sarcomas have been described in different parts of the body.[2]

Approximately 70% to 80% of HN sarcomas occur in adults; angiosarcoma, undifferentiated

Authors have nothing to disclose.
[a] Soft Tissue Pathology, Neuropathology and Autopsy Services, Department of Pathology and Laboratory Medicine, University of Florida College of Medicine, University of Florida, Jacksonville, 655 West 8th Street, Box C-504, Jacksonville, FL 32209-6511, USA; [b] Head and Neck Pathology, Department of Pathology and Laboratory Medicine, University of Florida College of Medicine, University of Florida, Jacksonville, 655 West 8th Street, Box C-504, Jacksonville, FL 32209-6511, USA; [c] Head and Neck Oncologic and Microvascular Surgery, Division of Head Neck Surgery, Department of Oral and Maxillofacial Surgery, University of Florida Health Science Center, Jacksonville, University of Florida College of Medicine, 653 West 8th Street, Jacksonville, FL 32209, USA; [d] Division of Surgical Oncology, University of Florida College of Medicine, 653 West 8th Street, Jacksonville, FL 32209, USA; [e] Head and Neck Oncologic Surgery and Microvascular Fellowship, Division of Head and Neck Surgery, Department of Oral and Maxillofacial Surgery, University of Florida Health Science Center, Jacksonville, University of Florida College of Medicine, 653 West 8th Street, Jacksonville, FL 32209, USA
* Corresponding author.
E-mail address: Arun.Gopinath@jax.ufl.edu

Oral Maxillofacial Surg Clin N Am 29 (2017) 355–366
http://dx.doi.org/10.1016/j.coms.2017.04.002
1042-3699/17/© 2017 Elsevier Inc. All rights reserved.

pleomorphic sarcoma (malignant fibrous histiocytoma), Kaposi sarcoma, and fibrosarcoma are the most common. Between 20% and 30% occur in children, with most being osteosarcoma, rhabdomyosarcoma and, EWS.[3]

PATHOGENESIS AND PREDISPOSING FACTORS IN HEAD AND NECK SARCOMAS

Several associated/predisposing factors have been implicated in the pathogenesis of bone and soft tissue sarcomas. These include genetic predisposition, acquired gene mutations, radiation/chemotherapy, chemical carcinogens, chronic irritation, lymphedema, viral infections, such as human immunodeficiency virus and human herpesvirus 8 in Kaposi sarcoma, and Epstein-Barr virus in smooth muscle tumors of immunocompromised patients.[4]

GENETIC PREDISPOSITION
Li-Fraumeni Syndrome

Li-Fraumeni syndrome (LFS) is an autosomal dominant inherited germline mutation in the p53 tumor suppressor gene. The syndrome is characterized by soft tissue and bone sarcomas, breast cancer, brain tumors, leukemia, and adrenocortical cancer before the age of 45 years. Sarcomas account for nearly 25% of tumors in affected individuals and they arise at a younger age than those unassociated with LFS.[5]

Retinoblastoma Gene

Different types of sarcomas develop later in life of patients irradiated for retinoblastoma from inherited mutant copy of retinoblastoma-1 gene. Some of these sarcomas did not arise within the irradiated field, suggesting that the gene mutation itself predisposes to secondary sarcomas with radiation therapy shortening the latent period and increasing the risk.[6]

Neurofibromatosis Type-I (Mutations in NF1 Gene)

Some of the multiple benign neurofibromas may transform to malignant peripheral nerve sheath tumor with complex karyotype. The malignant transformation is thought to reflect the 2-hit hypothesis in which one allele is constitutionally inactivated in the germline, and the other allele undergoes a "second hit" by complex molecular aberrations.[7]

Other than a genetic predisposition, acquired cytogenetic events in sarcomas fall into 2 major categories: those with specific genetic alterations that can be used to confirm the diagnosis, predict prognosis, or both,[8] and those with nonspecific complex genetic alterations, as in osteosarcoma, undifferentiated pleomorphic sarcoma (malignant fibrous histiocytoma), angiosarcoma, or leiomyosarcoma. A positive correlation exists between the genomic complexity and more aggressive tumor behavior.[9]

GENERAL PRINCIPLES IN DIAGNOSIS AND TREATMENT OF HEAD AND NECK SARCOMAS
Diagnosis

Patients present with symptoms driven by involvement of adjacent structures. Involvement of the skull base may produce diplopia, proptosis, facial pain, and headache. Involvement of the sinonasal tract may produce nasal obstruction, epistaxis, and pain. Larynx involvement may produce dysphonia or dyspnea. Computed tomography (CT) and MRI delineate the extent of bone and soft tissue involvement. Fludeoxyglucose-PET studies are performed when distant metastasis is suspected. Staging is performed according to American Joint Committee on Cancer guidelines. Open or core biopsy is essential for histologic diagnosis and grading. The tumors are histologically divided into 3 categories; low grade, intermediate grade, and high grade based on the Federation Nationale des Centers de Lutte Contre le Cancer grading system, which considers tumor differentiation, mitosis, and necrosis, and helps guide therapy.

Surgical Treatment

Complete surgical tumor resection with negative margins at the first attempt should be the prime objective to achieve local control, avoids the increased morbidity and costs of second surgery, and is the best chance for potential cure.

Classic teaching based largely on experience in non-HNS dictates the margins of tumor excision/resection may be classified as wide margin when a wide negative margin is present around the resected tumor, as a marginal excision when the excision plane passed through the reactive zone around the tumor (clear but close <1 mm), or an intralesional excision if the tumor is present at any part of the margins.[10]

An ideal "wide" resection margin may be difficult to achieve in HN sarcoma (HNS) without potential considerable functional morbidity from tumor proximity to vital HN structures. Therefore, in HNS, resection should be as wide as permitted by the nearby vital structures, which is commonly accepted clinically as a 1.0-cm thickness of uninvolved tissue around the mass, or an anatomic equivalent, such as periosteum, where appropriate.

Soft tissue sarcomas may deceptively appear grossly circumscribed. The presence of a plane of cleavage around some tumors allowing easy shelling out of the tumor may give a false impression of a benign or low-grade sarcoma and that excision was complete. Such "excisional biopsy" is suboptimal as the surrounding pseudocapsule is commonly infiltrated by tumor. Satellite foci are often present some distance from the main tumor and residual tumor will be identified on reexcision specimens.[11] Prior excisional biopsy makes it harder to achieve acceptable margins at the second reexcision attempt. Fascial planes have been disrupted and tumor spread is facilitated by wound hematoma, which makes it more difficult to accurately estimate the amount of residual tumor and which tissues have been contaminated by the first exposure. Imaging to assess the extent of residual tumor is of limited assistance because of postoperative changes in the bed of the original tumor.[12] Even when reexcision is histologically successful, there is often increased morbidity because of the need for more extensive surgery than is required for the initial resection, the extent of which cannot be determined accurately.

The incidence of lymph node metastases is sufficiently low in HNS that elective nodal dissection is not routinely indicated in absence of palpable nodes with few exceptions, as in angiosarcoma, epithelioid sarcoma, and rhabdomyosarcoma, in which nodal spread is not uncommon.[13]

Adjuvant Chemotherapy and Radiotherapy

Recommendations for adjuvant chemotherapy and/or radiation are made for each case based on multidisciplinary evaluation of all clinical and histopathologic features, tumor chemotherapy and radiation sensitivity, margins status, and high-risk conditions. Surgical excision combined with postoperative radiotherapy is the primary treatment for some types of sarcoma (as synovial sarcoma) even with negative resection margins. In other sarcomas, particularly rhabdomyosarcoma, the initial role of surgery may be limited to biopsy for diagnostic purposes and/or tumor debulking, depending on the patient.[14] In such cases, surgical or pathologic margin status is less of a concern, as multimodality therapy (combined chemotherapy, external-beam radiation, and nonradical surgery) is superior to any single-modality therapy of rhabdomyosarcoma.[14]

Variables with Possible Prognostic Impact in Head and Neck Sarcoma

Although histology and behavior of HNS is similar to their counterparts in other body sites,

comparative data for the overall survival rates are conflicting. Zagars and colleagues[15] studied the outcome in 1225 patients with soft tissue sarcomas in HN and non-HN locations treated between 1960 and 1999 with surgery and radiation therapy and found the 5-year local control rates and survival were inferior in HNS.

Another larger study using Surveillance, Epidemiology, and End Results (SEER) data on more than 12,000 patients with broad variety of HNS treated between 1973 and 2010 found 5-year survival figures comparable to non-HNS.[16]

Whether or not the location of HNS constitutes an independent risk factor for a worse prognosis appears unresolved. The inferior disease control is at least partially a function of the anatomic constraints for complete tumor resection rather than the difference in the biologic tumor behavior or histology. The tumor growth within the tight confines of the complex structural anatomy of the HN and its close proximity to vital structures are major obstacles limiting tumor resectability with adequate negative margins. The failure to obtain negative surgical margins is associated with failure of local control and a poor prognosis.[17]

In a series of 146 patients with a variety of skull base bone and soft tissue sarcomas, the 5-years survival rates were 77%, 43%, and 36% with negative, marginal (<1 mm), and positive surgical margins, respectively. The presence of positive or close margin was an independent predictor of poor survival in multivariate analysis.[18]

The main cause of death from HNS is progressive local recurrence before distant metastatic spread. The main cause of death from non-HNS is the widespread tumor metastasis. In a study on 103 patients with HNS treated from 1944 to 1988, local recurrence was the sole cause of death in 63% of cases.[19] These data emphasize the adverse prognostic impact of positive resection margins in HNS. Other important prognostic factors include male gender, tumor histologic grade, size, stage, nodal status, and prior radiation in multivariate analysis of the SEER database.[16]

The prognosis is adversely affected by the tumor size and histologic grade. Park and colleagues[13] reviewed 122 cases of HNS, and determined that high histologic grade was associated with significantly worse patient survival when compared with low-grade sarcomas. In addition, locoregional recurrence rates were much higher for lesions measuring larger than 10 cm in diameter when compared with tumors of 5 cm or smaller.

Prognosis also may be affected by the histologic subtype of sarcoma identified. Results from the Head and Neck Sarcoma Registry of the Society of Head and Neck Surgeons on 214 patients with HNS (194 adults and 20 children) identified the major determinants of survival were adequacy of resection margins and histologic type. The survival was near 100% in patients with CS or dermatofibrosarcoma protuberans compared with 60% to 70% with malignant fibrous histiocytoma or fibrosarcoma. The worst survival (<50% at 5 years) was with osteosarcoma, angiosarcoma, rhabdomyosarcoma, and malignant peripheral nerve sheath tumor associated with NF1.[17]

Most published sarcoma series report outcomes involving cases over several decades, given the rarity of HNS. Reporting results in this manner often fails to reflect diagnostic refinements, and possible impact in outcomes achieved with the advance in diagnostic tools, surgical techniques, and chemo/radiotherapy management of sarcomas. As an example, rhabdomyosarcoma, which was rarely cured before the modern chemotherapy and combined modality approaches, is now curable in more than 80% of children.[20]

Although lymph node metastases may be regarded an essential part of staging, lymph node metastases in HNS is uncommon, occurring in approximately 10% of cases and most commonly from rhabdomyosarcoma and angiosarcoma of the scalp.[2] The data on the prognostic impact of nodal metastases are conflicting.[21,22]

Postirradiation sarcomas of the HN are associated with a poor prognosis when compared with sarcomas not induced by irradiation. The poor outcome in postradiation sarcomas may be attributed to the high histologic grade and aggressive nature of most of radiation-induced sarcomas and the limited ability to give full-dose radiotherapy to a site that has been previously irradiated. Additionally, the use of prior chemotherapy for the first cancer may limit choices for subsequent therapy. The alterations and scarring in the radiated field may compromise the ability to successfully resect a tumor with wide surgical margins.[23]

RESECTION MARGINS AFFECT RECURRENCE RATE AND TREATMENT MODALITIES IN SELECTED HEAD AND NECK SARCOMA
Osteosarcoma

Fewer than 10% of osteosarcomas in the body occur in the HN, with a median age of 10 to 20 years older than osteosarcoma of long bones. The most common site in HN is maxilla and mandible and rarely calvaria.[24] Osteosarcoma may arise secondary to radiotherapy (**Fig. 1**) or Paget disease. Primary osteosarcoma may have genetic predisposition as mutation of TP53 tumor

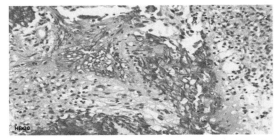

Fig. 1. Radiation-induced osteosarcoma in the mandible developing after irradiation of squamous cell carcinoma of tonsil. HE, hematoxylin-eosin.

suppressor gene in LFS, retinoblastoma gene, or heterogeneous genetic complexity.[5,6,9]

On plain film, the classic features include destructive lytic or sclerotic tumor. "Sunburst" and "hair-on-end" appearance on the tumor surface result from rapid tumor growth causing stretching and perpendicular ossification of Sharpey fibers connecting the periosteum to bone. Also, a triangular area of new subperiosteal bone, referred as "Codman triangle," is created when the tumor raises the periosteum away from the bone. In addition, widening of the periodontal ligament, known as "Garrington sign," may be seen on panoramic radiograph.[2,24]

Osteosarcoma is classified according to the location into medullary (within the bone), from bone surface (parosteal and periosteal) or rarely extraosseous. Grossly, the tumor may appear soft (osteolytic) or sclerotic (osteosclerotic), depending on the degree of mineralization. Histology is characterized by malignant osteoid (precursor of bone) within a sarcomatous spindle to round anaplastic stromal cells. According to the predominant stromal component, osteosarcoma can be subtyped as osteoblastic/osteosclerotic, chondroblastic, fibroblastic, giant cell–rich, small cell, epithelioid, and telangiectatic (**Fig. 2**). Histologic grades range from low to high grade based on the degree of cellular atypia/anaplasia and mitoses.[2]

Management of head and neck osteosarcoma
Tumor resection with wide clear margins at the first attempt is critical for local control and potential complete cure. The definition of wide, clear margins is consistently defined in the literature. Fernandes and colleagues[24] recommended a 3-cm clinically clear margin, as recurrence was reported with less than 1-cm negative margin. This may be difficult in maxilla or skull base tumors, and 43% of resected sarcomas at these sites have demonstrated positive margins.[18] Granados-Garcia and colleagues[25] note that cases in which total

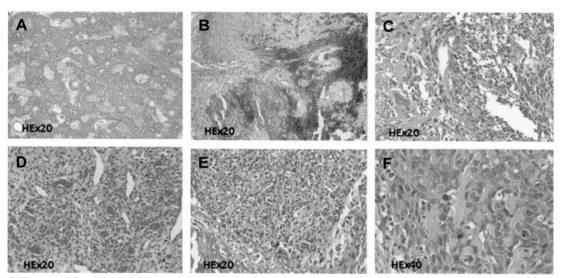

Fig. 2. Osteosarcoma with malignant osteoid matrix ranging from dense sclerosis to thin lacy osteoid trabeculae. Histologic subtypes: osteosclerotic (*A*), chondroblastic (*B*), fibroblastic (*C*), giant cell–rich (*D*), small cell (E), and epithelioid (*F*).

mandibulectomy was performed did not show improved local control or survival benefit when compared with segmental mandibular resection. Soft tissue invasion was hypothesized as the source of local failure, although the status of the soft tissue margin was not clearly stated.[25] More recently, Vassiliou and colleagues[26] highlight their practice of hemi-mandibulectomy with condylar disarticulation in cases of osteosarcoma with radiographic extension to the ramus.

The benefits of adjuvant chemo/radiotherapy have been controversial. Osteosarcomas are relatively resistant to radiation therapy with insignificant effect as a primary modality. However, radiotherapy is considered to reduce local recurrence and improve overall survival for patients with positive/uncertain surgical margins.[27,28]

A small study on 15 cases did not show significant benefit from neoadjuvant chemotherapy.[29] In contrast, another study on 36 cases of HN osteosarcoma found that combined surgery/neoadjuvant chemotherapy improved the 2-year and 5-year survival rates compared with surgery alone.[30] In select patients, neoadjuvant chemotherapy may decrease the burden of unresectable tumors, and in cases with unfavorable histopathologic findings, the addition of chemotherapy may improve local control.[31]

Chondrosarcoma

Approximately 5% to 10% of CSs are located in the HN, with predilection for larynx, followed by maxilla, mandible, and skull base. CT and MR

are the preferred imaging modalities to delineate the tumor, calcifications, and extent of bone and soft tissue invasion.[2]

Grossly, CSs are usually ≥3 cm, lobular, white to bluish, with firm or myxoid to gelatinous consistency. Histologically, CS is formed of atypical/malignant chondrocytes in hyaline/myxoid matrix with no osteoid formation. Calcification may be present. Histologic grades of CS range from well-differentiated (grade 1) to poorly differentiated (grade III) or dedifferentiated based on tumor cellularity, atypia/anaplasia, and number of mitoses (**Fig. 3**).

Most CSs are well-differentiated; grades II and III are associated with a poorer prognosis.[2] Myxoid CS (mimicking small round blue cell tumors) and mesenchymal CS (mimicking solitary fibrous tumor) are other less common variants.

Surgical resection with negative margins is the gold treatment standard. The type of resection depends on the tumor location/extension and histologic grade. Complete resection of skull base tumors may be impossible, and decompression of vital structures with tumor debulking may be the available option followed by adjuvant radiotherapy or close observation. For laryngeal tumors, the surgical approach may be conservative for low-grade tumors. Local recurrence is present in approximately 50% of patients, particularly with conservation surgery. Given the low rate of nodal metastases, neck dissection is not recommended. Total laryngectomy is recommended for high-grade tumors.[32] There are no clear, consistent recommended criteria in

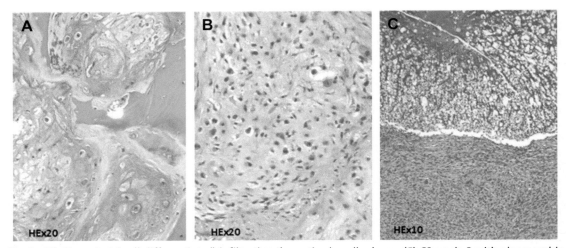

Fig. 3. (*A*) CS grade 1 (well-differentiated) infiltrating the native lamellar bone. (*B*) CS grade 3 with pleomorphic malignant chondrocytes. (*C*) Dedifferentiated CS showing sharp transition of cartilaginous tumor to undifferentiated sarcoma.

the literature for the "optimal surgical margins" in CS.

CSs are relatively resistant to radiotherapy, and chemotherapy is of uncertain benefit in low-grade CS due to the low fraction of dividing cells. However, adjuvant radiation and in select cases, chemotherapy are recommended for aggressive, high-grade CSs, residual disease, or palliative for unresectable tumors.[32,33]

Rhabdomyosarcoma

Rhabdomyosarcoma (RMS) is a sarcoma of skeletal muscle, predominantly affecting children. Up to 40% of cases occur in the HN.[34]

Grossly, RMS is soft to fleshy and varies according to the location from large polypoid, multinodular, or grapelike (termed sarcoma botryoides) in nasopharynx or sinonasal tract or small aural polyp in ear to orbital/lid mass.[2]

Histologic subtypes of RMS include embryonal, alveolar, pleomorphic, sclerosing, and mixed. RMS is characterized by immunoreactivity to markers of skeletal muscle differentiation like desmin, myogenin, and Myo D1, which are helpful in diagnosis as well as pathologic margin evaluation (**Fig. 4**).

Embryonal subtype is the most common (>70%), with a better prognosis, and pleomorphic RMS is the least common and is more common in

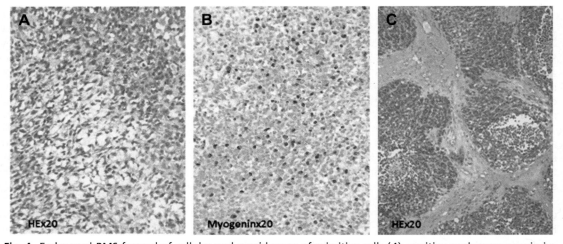

Fig. 4. Embryonal RMS formed of cellular and myoid areas of primitive cells (*A*), positive nuclear myogenin immunostain (*B*), alveolar RMS characterized by nests/sheets of poorly differentiated tumor cells with central necrosis, loss of cellular cohesion, and surrounding hyalinized fibrous septa (*C*).

older patients. Alveolar RMS is characterized by the genetic translocations PAX3/7-FKHR (FOXO1) and has a poorer prognosis.[2]

Treatment and prognosis

The distinction between parameningeal and nonparameningeal RMS has important reflection on prognosis and treatment. Up to 40% of HN RMSs are parameningeal in close proximity to the nasopharynx, nasal cavity, paranasal sinuses, middle ear, mastoid, and infratemporal and pterygopalatine fossa preventing complete tumor resection without unacceptable morbidity. In addition, these tumors have increased propensity for meningeal extension, a fatal pattern of progression with high-risk cranial nerve palsy, skull base invasion, and intracranial extension.[35]

Complete surgical resection with negative margins whenever possible is the ideal treatment; however, the width of the recommended surgical margin remains undefined. Surgical excision with the expectation of a negative pathologic margin is often not feasible in HN and, in many cases, the initial role of surgery is limited to biopsy diagnosis and/or tumor debulking surgery (DS). A recent study reported that no significant improvement in patient outcome was associated with DS when compared with biopsy sampling surgery, although DS may have a palliative role, and offers an opportunity remove necrotic or malodorous tissue.[14]

Routine nodal dissection is considered unnecessary unless recommended from clinical/radiographic screening, particularly in parameningeal rhabdomyosarcoma and alveolar histology, which has a higher risk for nodal dissemination and increased mortality.[36]

Ewing sarcoma

Primary EWS of HN is extremely rare, comprising approximately 4% to 9% of all EWS with a peak incidence in the first 2 decades of life. The most common primary sites are the skull, maxilla, and mandible.[37]

The typical radiographic appearance of EWS is a permeative destruction of bone associated with a large soft tissue mass. Periosteal reaction with the characteristic onion-skin lamination or vertical spiculation is uncommon.[38]

Histologic diagnosis of EWS may be difficult to differentiate from other small blue cell tumors. However, in more than 90% of cases, the tumor cells demonstrate characteristic/diagnostic translocation between chromosomes 11 and 22 (t [11;22] [q24;q12]) (**Fig. 5**).[2]

Treatment and prognosis

The prognosis of EWS in HN is adversely affected by the patient age, disease stage, and tumor volume at diagnosis. A multidisciplinary approach with surgery, radiotherapy, and chemotherapy or a combination is critical in the management of EWS. EWS treatment often begins with induction chemotherapy followed by surgical removal with negative margins where possible. Multimodality therapy has dramatically improved the 5-year survival to more than 70% for localized disease in the HN. However, minimal long-term follow-up is available for HN EWS. Surgery should be combined with radiotherapy in case of marginal resection and/or poor histologic response.[37] Similar to other HNS, the optimal clinical margin recommended for adequate surgical excision has not been identified in the literature.

Liposarcoma

Liposarcoma is one of the most common soft tissue sarcomas in the body, but liposarcoma in the head and neck region is uncommon.[39] Only 3% to 9% of liposarcomas occur in the HN, mainly the subcutaneous region of the neck and cheek.[39] Liposarcoma may clinically appear encapsulated or well demarcated. However, infiltrating borders are common at microscopic evaluation. Numerous histologic variants exist: well-differentiated, intermediate-grade lesions including myxoid/round cell liposarcoma and high-grade variants, such as pleomorphic and dedifferentiated types (**Fig. 6**). Well-differentiated variants, including lipomalike, sclerosing, and inflammatory subtypes, are distinguished from reactive or benign adipocytic lesions by CDK4 positivity (see **Fig. 6**A–C) and MDM2 amplification.[2]

Liposarcomas of HN are usually early stage at diagnosis, low grade, and with fewer nodal metastases and significantly better prognosis than in other body sites.[39] Resection with wide margins is important to encompass the microscopic infiltration despite the apparent gross encapsulation. Definitive resection margin status can be challenging to determine in some cases, particularly well-differentiated tumors with margins placed in regional adipose tissue. In one study, margin data were not available for review in nearly 60% of patients, although the tumor grade and margin status were not clearly stated.[40] A recent review of patients with HN liposarcoma noted the disease-specific survival for patients with HN liposarcoma treated with single-modality radiation therapy was lower than for the group of patients treated surgically or by combined surgery/radiation therapy.[39] A similar pattern was also observed

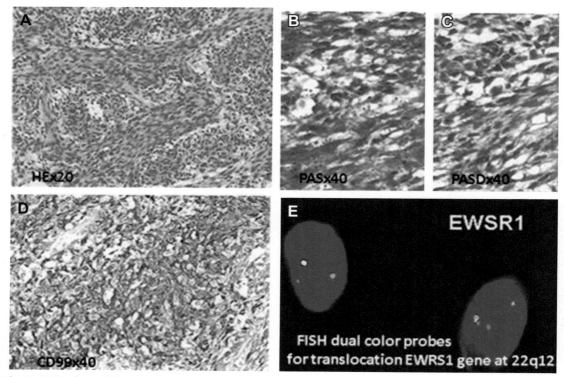

Fig. 5. EWS of mandible showing compact short fascicles of spindle cells blending with hyperchromatic round cells (*A*). Vacuolated cytoplasm containing periodic acid-Schiff–positive, diastase labile glycogen granules (*B*, *C*). Strong CD99 membranous positivity in the tumor cells (*D*). Fluorescence in situ hybridization showing yellow or red–green fusion of EWS-FLI1 gene signals consistent with positive translocation for EWS/primitive neuroectodermal tumor (*E*).

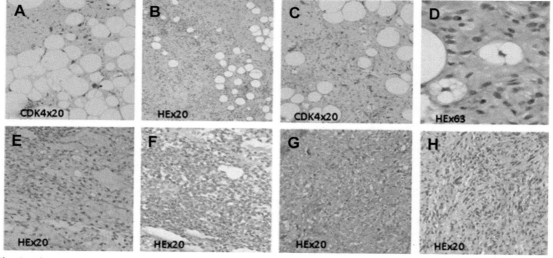

Fig. 6. Diagnostic CDk4-positive atypical cells in well-differentiated lipomalike (*A*) and inflammatory liposarcoma (*B, C*) with characteristic lipoblasts (*D*). Myxoid liposarcoma (*E*) with round cell transformation (*F*), pleomorphic liposarcoma (*G*), and dedifferentiated liposarcoma into undifferentiated pleomorphic sarcoma (*H*).

for rates of overall survival, with a trend toward survival benefit in the surgery-alone cohort.[39]

Angiosarcoma

Angiosarcomas (ASs) are uncommon, aggressive tumors of blood or lymphatic vessels and account for approximately 1% of all sarcomas.[4] More than half of ASs occur in the HN, mainly the scalp and face, and therefore potentially amenable to complete resection.[41]

Grossly, AS ranges from red-purple, painless papules/nodules to extensively ulcerated locally infiltrative mass. Tumor histology ranges from well-differentiated, but intercommunicating invasive, vascular spaces to high-grade poorly differentiated solid pleomorphic cellularity expressing vascular endothelial markers as CD31, erg, and Factor VIII (**Fig. 7**).

Radical surgery with negative margins is not feasible in most cases because of the multifocal nature and extensive local, microscopic spread in AS. Multiple mapping biopsies as a method to define the extent of AS has been attempted by some, but would likely be subject to sampling bias and is no guarantee for negative surgical margins.[42,43] A retrospective study by Patel and colleagues[41] of patients with AS of the face or scalp showed a better response to multimodal therapy (combination of surgery with lymph node dissection, radiation, and/or chemotherapy) than to individual treatments alone.

Synovial Sarcoma

Synovial sarcoma (SS) in HN is an extremely rare aggressive high-grade sarcoma, affecting mainly the neck, hypopharynx, and retropharynx thought to arise from primitive mesenchymal cells, unrelated to synovial membranes or synovial tissue.[44] The tumor histology displays epithelial, spindle cell, or combined biphasic morphology. SS has a distinctive immunostain profile and TLE-1 nuclear staining is sensitive and specific marker for SS (**Fig. 8**).

The diagnosis is confirmed by the characteristic translocation t(x,18).[2] Local recurrence rates are high (60%–90%) due to the limited resectability in some HN locations. Treatment should be directed toward complete surgical resection. Review of one recent series of 15 cases demonstrates the formidable surgical challenge of HN SS, with approximately half the cases resected to negative margins. In this series, no patient with clear margins experienced recurrence, whereas 44% of the patients with positive resection margins recurred, and patients with recurrent disease were found to have a reduction in survival.[44]

In contrast, at least 2 studies have not been able to identify a significant relationship with surgical margin status and overall survival.[45,46] In the more recent study, only tumor recurrence was associated with an effect on disease-specific survival,[46] prompting the recommendation for consideration of multimodality therapy in patients with large tumors (>5 cm) and anatomic sites challenging to access.[45,46] Given the aggressive behavior and infiltrative pattern of growth, excision with wide surgical margins is an important component to reduce local recurrence. Nonetheless, a multimodality approach, especially in high-risk patients, is often used to reduce the rate of local recurrence.[45]

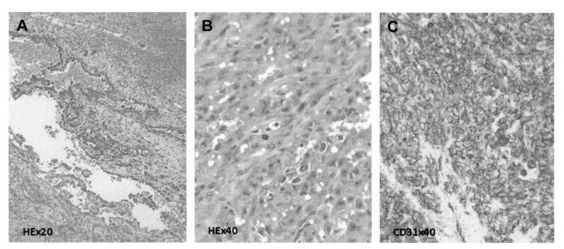

Fig. 7. Intercommunicating invasive vascular spaces (*A*), solid growth of epithelioid malignant cells with poorly formed vascular clefts (*B*) positive for CD31 vascular endothelial marker (*C*).

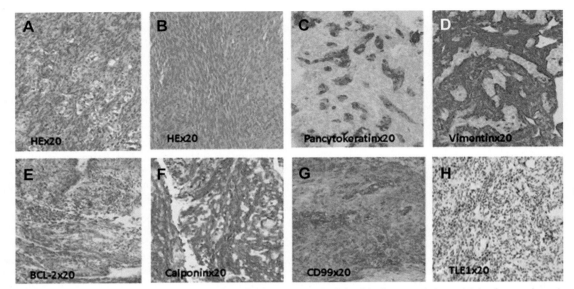

Fig. 8. SS, biphasic epithelial (*A*) and spindle cell (*B*) components (*A*) with characteristic positivity for cytokeratin in the epithelial cells (*C*), vimentin in spindle cells (*D*), BCL2 (*E*), calponin (*F*), CD99 (*G*), and TLE1sensitive and specific for SS (*H*).

Fibrosarcoma

Fibrosarcomas account for 12% to 19% of soft tissue sarcomas. Approximately 10% occur in the HN, mainly in sinonasal tract, neck, and jaw. Fibrosarcomas may be a late complication of radiation therapy or burn injury. Most cases occur between 30 and 60 years of age. An infantile variant occurs in those younger than 2 years and has a better prognosis [14]. Grossly, fibrosarcomas appear firm, tan-gray, and well-circumscribed, but microscopically invasive. Histologically, most are well-differentiated, and characterized by fascicular or herringbone pattern of uniform spindle cells with tapered nuclei and variable collagen production (**Fig. 9**).

Poorly differentiated or high-grade fibrosarcoma have cellular pleomorphism, hyperchromatism, frequent mitosis, scant collagen, tumor necrosis, and hemorrhage. Fibrosarcomas are largely nonreactive to immunostains (except vimentin), distinguishing it from other spindle cell sarcomas.

A series of 29 patients with HN fibrosarcoma treated at UCLA Medical Center showed that tumor grade is the most important prognostic factor, followed by tumor size (>5 cm) and surgical margin status. The study recommended surgical resection alone with adequate margin for low-grade fibrosarcoma and postoperative adjuvant radiotherapy for high-grade tumors or positive surgical margins. Significant limitations of this series include retrospective data collected over a 30-year period with details lacking as to what constitutes an adequate surgical negative margin.[47,48]

SUMMARY

HN sarcomas are rare and can present management difficulties. These tumors are best managed in a multidisciplinary setting. Tumor resection with clear surgical margins, although the treatment of choice, may not be possible due to the anatomic constraints in HN. In most patients, except those with small resectable low-grade lesions, adjuvant radiotherapy and chemotherapy is added to maximize local control with variable results according to the tumor sensitivity.

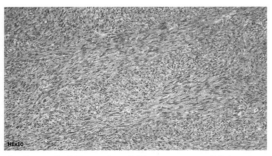

Fig. 9. Well-differentiated fibrosarcoma with herringbone pattern of malignant spindle cells.

REFERENCES

1. O'Neill JP, Bilsky MH, Kraus D. Head and neck sarcomas: epidemiology, pathology, and management. Neurosurg Clin N Am 2013;24(1):67–78.

2. Fletcher CD, Bridge JA, Hogendoorn PCW, et al. WHO classification of soft tissue and bone tumors. 4th edition. Lyon (France): IARC press; 2013.

3. Potter BO, Sturgis EM. Sarcomas of the head and neck. Surg Oncol Clin N Am 2003;12(2):379–417.

4. Zahm SH, Fraumeni JF Jr. The epidemiology of soft tissue sarcoma. Semin Oncol 1997;24(5):504–14.

5. Ognjanovic S, Olivier M, Bergemann TL, et al. Sarcomas in TP53 germline mutation carriers: a review of the IARC TP53 database. Cancer 2012;118(5): 1387–96.

6. Kleinerman RA, Tucker MA, Abramson DH, et al. Risk of soft tissue sarcomas by individual subtype in survivors of hereditary retinoblastoma. J Natl Cancer Inst 2007;99(1):24–31.

7. Farid M, Demicco EG, Garcia R, et al. Malignant peripheral nerve sheath tumors. Oncologist 2014; 19(2):193–201.

8. Italiano A, Di Mauro I, Rapp J, et al. Clinical effect of molecular methods in sarcoma diagnosis (GENSARC): a prospective, multicentre, observational study. Lancet Oncol 2016;17(4):532–8.

9. Chibon F, Lagarde P, Salas S, et al. Validated prediction of clinical outcome in sarcomas and multiple types of cancer on the basis of a gene expression signature related to genome complexity. Nat Med 2010;16(7):781–7.

10. Rydholm A. Surgical margins for soft tissue sarcoma. Acta Orthop Scand Suppl 1997;273:81–5.

11. Enneking WF, Spanier SS, Malawer MM. The effect of the anatomic setting on the results of surgical procedures for soft parts sarcoma of the thigh. Cancer 1981;47(5):1005–22.

12. Hudson TM, Schakel M, Springfield DS. Limitations of computed tomography following excisional biopsy of soft tissue sarcomas. Skeletal Radiol 1985; 13(1):49–54.

13. Park JT, Roh JL, Kim SO, et al. Prognostic factors and oncological outcomes of 122 head and neck soft tissue sarcoma patients treated at a single institution. Ann Surg Oncol 2015;22(1):248–55.

14. Cecchetto G, Bisogno G, De Corti F, et al. Biopsy or debulking surgery as initial surgery for locally advanced rhabdomyosarcomas in children? The experience of the Italian Cooperative Group studies. Cancer 2007;110(11):2561–7.

15. Zagars GK, Ballo MT, Pisters PW, et al. Prognostic factors for patients with localized soft-tissue sarcoma treated with conservation surgery and radiation therapy: an analysis of 1225 patients. Cancer 2003;97(10):2530–43.

16. Peng KA, Grogan T, Wang MB. Head and neck sarcomas: analysis of the SEER database. Otolaryngol Head Neck Surg 2014;151(4):627–33.

17. Wanebo HJ, Koness RJ, MacFarlane JK, et al. Head and neck sarcoma: report of the Head and Neck Sarcoma Registry. Society of Head and Neck Surgeons Committee on Research. Head Neck 1992;14(1):1–7.

18. Gil Z, Patel SG, Singh B, et al. Analysis of prognostic factors in 146 patients with anterior skull base sarcoma: an international collaborative study. Cancer 2007;110(5):1033–41.

19. Eeles RA, Fisher C, A'Hern RP, et al. Head and neck sarcomas: prognostic factors and implications for treatment. Br J Cancer 1993;68(1):201–7.

20. Pappo AS, Meza JL, Donaldson SS, et al. Treatment of localized nonorbital, nonparameningeal head and neck rhabdomyosarcoma: lessons learned from intergroup rhabdomyosarcoma studies III and IV. J Clin Oncol 2003;21(4):638–45.

21. Smith VA, Overton LJ, Lentsch EJ. Head and neck soft tissue sarcomas: unique lack of significance of synchronous node metastases. J Surg Oncol 2012; 106(7):837–43.

22. de Bree R, van der Valk P, Kuik DJ, et al. Prognostic factors in adult soft tissue sarcomas of the head and neck: a single-centre experience. Oral Oncol 2006; 42(7):703–9.

23. Yeang MS, Tay K, Ong WS, et al. Outcomes and prognostic factors of post-irradiation and de novo sarcomas of the head and neck: a histologically matched case-control study. Ann Surg Oncol 2013; 20(9):3066–75.

24. Fernandes R, Nikitakis NG, Pazoki A, et al. Osteogenic sarcoma of the jaw: a 10-year experience. J Oral Maxillofac Surg 2007;65(7):1286–91.

25. Granados-Garcia M, Luna-Ortiz K, Castillo-Oliva HA, et al. Free osseous and soft tissue surgical margins as prognostic factors in mandibular osteosarcoma. Oral Oncol 2006;42(2):172–6.

26. Vassiliou LV, Lalabekyan B, Jay A, et al. Head and neck sarcomas: a single institute series. Oral Oncol 2017;65:16–22.

27. Guadagnolo BA, Zagars GK, Raymond AK, et al. Osteosarcoma of the jaw/craniofacial region: outcomes after multimodality treatment. Cancer 2009; 115(14):3262–70.

28. Chen Y, Shen Q, Gokavarapu S, et al. Osteosarcoma of head and neck: a retrospective study on prognostic factors from a single institute database. Oral Oncol 2016;58:1–7.

29. DeAngelis AF, Spinou C, Tsui A, et al. Outcomes of patients with maxillofacial osteosarcoma: a review of 15 cases. J Oral Maxillofac Surg 2012;70(3): 734–9.

30. Mucke T, Mitchell DA, Tannapfel A, et al. Effect of neoadjuvant treatment in the management of osteosarcomas of the head and neck. J Cancer Res Clin Oncol 2014;140(1):127–31.

31. Smeele LE, Kostense PJ, van der Waal I, et al. Effect of chemotherapy on survival of craniofacial osteosarcoma: a systematic review of 201 patients. J Clin Oncol 1997;15(1):363–7.

32. Chin OY, Dubal PM, Sheikh AB, et al. Laryngeal chondrosarcoma: a systematic review of 592 cases. Laryngoscope 2017;127(2):430–9.

33. Coca-Pelaz A, Rodrigo JP, Triantafyllou A, et al. Chondrosarcomas of the head and neck. Eur Arch Otorhinolaryngol 2014;271(10):2601–9.

34. Radzikowska J, Kukwa W, Kukwa A, et al. Rhabdomyosarcoma of the head and neck in children. Contemp Oncol (Pozn) 2015;19(2):98–107.

35. Tefft M, Fernandez C, Donaldson M, et al. Incidence of meningeal involvement by rhabdomyosarcoma of the head and neck in children: a report of the Intergroup Rhabdomyosarcoma Study (IRS). Cancer 1978;42(1):253–8.

36. Terwisscha van Scheltinga CE, Spronk P, van Rosmalen J, et al. Diagnosis and treatment of lymph node metastases in pediatric rhabdomyosarcoma in the Netherlands: a retrospective analysis. J Pediatr Surg 2014;49(3):416–9.

37. Grevener K, Haveman LM, Ranft A, et al. Management and outcome of Ewing sarcoma of the head and neck. Pediatr Blood Cancer 2016;63(4):604–10.

38. Mar WA, Taljanovic MS, Bagatell R, et al. Update on imaging and treatment of Ewing sarcoma family tumors: what the radiologist needs to know. J Comput Assist Tomogr 2008;32(1):108–18.

39. Gerry D, Fox NF, Spruill LS, et al. Liposarcoma of the head and neck: analysis of 318 cases with comparison to non-head and neck sites. Head Neck 2014; 36(3):393–400.

40. Davis EC, Ballo MT, Luna MA, et al. Liposarcoma of the head and neck: The University of Texas M. D. Anderson Cancer Center experience. Head Neck 2009;31(1):28–36.

41. Patel SH, Hayden RE, Hinni ML, et al. Angiosarcoma of the scalp and face: the Mayo Clinic experience. JAMA Otolaryngol Head Neck Surg 2015;141(4): 335–40.

42. Bullen R, Larson PO, Landeck AE, et al. Angiosarcoma of the head and neck managed by a combination of multiple biopsies to determine tumor margin and radiation therapy. Report of three cases and review of the literature. Dermatol Surg 1998;24(10): 1105–10.

43. Harati K, Daigeler A, Goertz O, et al. Primary and secondary soft tissue angiosarcomas: prognostic significance of surgical margins in 43 patients. Anticancer Res 2016;36(8):4321–8.

44. Salcedo-Hernandez RA, Lino-Silva LS, Luna-Ortiz K. Synovial sarcomas of the head and neck: comparative analysis with synovial sarcoma of the extremities. Auris Nasus Larynx 2013; 40(5):476–80.

45. Harb WJ, Luna MA, Patel SR, et al. Survival in patients with synovial sarcoma of the head and neck: association with tumor location, size, and extension. Head Neck 2007;29(8):731–40.

46. Owosho AA, Estilo CL, Rosen EB, et al. A clinicopathologic study on SS18 fusion positive head and neck synovial sarcomas. Oral Oncol 2017;66:46–51.

47. Mark RJ, Sercarz JA, Tran L, et al. Fibrosarcoma of the head and neck. The UCLA experience. Arch Otolaryngol Head Neck Surg 1991;117: 396–401.

48. Tran LM, Mark R, Meier R, et al. Sarcomas of the head and neck. Prognostic factors and tretament strategies. Cancer 1992;70:169–77.

Surgical Margins
The Perspective of Pathology

Kelly R. Magliocca, DDS, MPH

KEYWORDS

- Surgical margins • Gross examination • Histopathologic examination • Squamous cell carcinoma
- Indeterminate margin status

KEY POINTS

- Clear communication between the surgical and pathology team members is essential for optimal understanding of the resection specimen.
- Although tumor extension from deeper margin tissues may be more challenging to access, information from all surgical margin types is important in evaluating and achieving 3-dimensional margin clearance.
- The manner in which post-removal specimen alterations impact the relationship of tumor to surgical margins remains understudied.

OVERVIEW

Neoplasms of the head and neck constitute a broad spectrum of benign and malignant entities. When the treatment plan involves resection, assessment of the surgical margins represents an important component of the pathologic examination and margin status is regarded as an important indicator of a complete surgical resection. In the head and neck, much of the literature pertaining to surgical margins is dedicated to mucosal squamous cell carcinoma (mSCCa) and cutaneous malignancy, with less study performed on other disease processes or conditions. The ability to generalize conclusions such as 'safe distance' measurements from work performed in mSCCa or cutaneous malignancy to other types of neoplasms in the head and neck region seems limited, and the importance of margin status is best studied within each disease type. That aside, there remains the daily practice of surgery and the daily practice of pathology, and this article is intended to review conditions and considerations that may impact reliable margin assessment and interpretation.

THE HANDOFF ORIENTATION

The 'handoff' orientation refers to the face-to-face meeting between the surgeon and pathologist to review the surgical specimen characteristics. Though there is little in the way of peer reviewed literature upon which to evaluate advantages, disadvantages, timing or nature of the handoff orientation and/or impact on final margin status, anecdotes and interdisciplinary teaching suggests the practice helps to minimize ambiguity in margin determination. In some large or multi-campus institutions, surgeons and pathologists may not be located in the same place, however, when both teams are present, the handoff orientation can occur simultaneously with a specimen-based frozen section request, or at the conclusion of the surgical procedure. Handoff orientation may be less satisfying when performed on formalin-fixed specimen as the original specimen color, tissue texture, pliability and subtle specimen clues are irreversibly altered by fixation and may be less familiar appearing to the surgical team. In the ideal situation, specimen review occurs in the pathology suite to facilitate ready access to inking,

Department of Pathology and Laboratory Medicine, Emory University, Atlanta, GA 30322, USA
E-mail address: kmagliocca@emory.edu

Oral Maxillofacial Surg Clin N Am 29 (2017) 367–375
http://dx.doi.org/10.1016/j.coms.2017.05.002
1042-3699/17/© 2017 Elsevier Inc. All rights reserved.

disposable supplies, paperwork for notation of landmarks and measurements, and many times the involvement of more than the pathology departmental representative (eg, physician assistant, pathologist, pathology resident, or fellow). The handoff, regardless of specimen complexity, provides an opportunity for interdisciplinary communication and is encouraged whenever possible.[1] Highlighting anatomic components,

substation levels of an in-continuity cervical neck dissection, measurement of tumor in the unfixed state, agreement regarding identification and naming conventions of surgical margins, gross assessment of margins, and identification of areas of concern the surgeon would like to have further evaluated by frozen section represent possible elements for discussion (**Fig. 1**). Establishing which tissue surfaces represent specimen margins, in

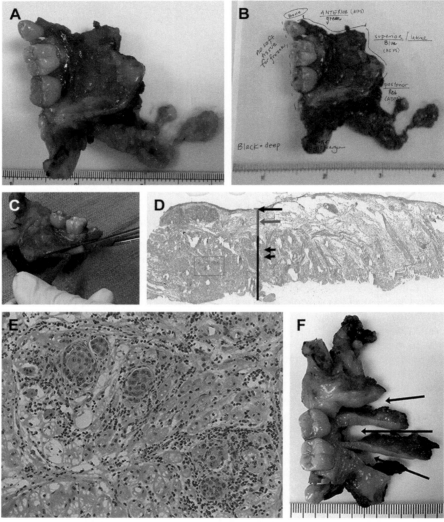

Fig. 1. Recurrent mucosal squamous cell carcinoma of buccal mucosa. Fresh resection specimen submitted for frozen section (FS) evaluation, before inking (*A*), photograph of specimen provides map of mucosal margins sampled from resection specimen, (perpendicular margin sampling map/notation not shown) (*B*), mucosal margin removed by physician assistant from main specimen (*C*), histologic layers of this mucosal margin includes: oral surface epithelium (*single black arrow*), subepithelial stroma (*blue arrow*), and skeletal muscle (*double black arrow*). Although not grossly visible, an isolated focus of infiltrating squamous cell carcinoma is identified in the skeletal muscle layer (*green box*) (stain: hematoxylin and eosin [H&E]; original magnification, ×4) (*D*), higher magnification of infiltrating squamous cell carcinoma in skeletal muscle (stain: H&E; original magnification, ×200) (*E*), appearance of fresh resection specimen (compare to picture A) after removal of 360 degree mucosal margins and 3 areas of tumor sampled in relation to the underlying deep soft tissue margin at the time of FS evaluation (*black arrows*) (*F*).

addition to naming conventions of the margins enhances communication between the pathology and surgical teams, and could facilitate surgical relocalization of a problematic area if the need arises. The specimen should be blotted dry for the handoff examination and before the application of ink, and observed for pooling or seepage of mucinous, clear, keratinous-appearing material or hemorrhagic accumulations. These findings may represent key areas to sample from the main specimen, particularly in cystic, myxoid, or mucinous salivary gland neoplasms, and cystic or myxoid odontogenic tumors (**Fig. 2**). In cases of nonneoplastic disease, such as soft tissue cysts or odontogenic cysts, there may be circumstances under which documentation of specimen integrity and absence of cyst wall disruption is of interest to the submitting surgeon, and this gross examination is best performed on fresh, unfixed specimens at the time of handoff.

Gnathic resections performed in the management of osteomyelitis or osteonecrosis range in specimen complexity and may include bone in several fragments owing to preexisting pathologic fracture, or multiple bone segments with multiple straight bone cuts, indicating possible bone margins. In cases where a cut surface of the mandible is suspected to be non-viable, additional surgical excision of sequential mandibular segments will be removed until bleeding bone is encountered. Submission of multiple bone fragments exhibiting a straight surgical saw-blade cut appearance (possible bone margin?) within the same specimen cup but without orientation undermines the ability of the pathology team to identify the true margin (**Fig. 3**). In addition to bone and/or soft tissue,

mucosal surfaces and facial skin removed surrounding an oral-cutaneous fistula may be present and necessitate microscopic evaluation of these inked margin types. In most surgical specimens however, significant fragmentation precludes margin analysis. Patients undergoing bone resection for osteo(radio)necrosis may have a history of primary oral cavity or oropharyngeal malignancy or a history of metastatic carcinoma, such as breast or prostate cancer; therefore mucosal, skin, and bone margin sampling, even for resections performed for presumed nonneoplastic gnathic disease, is an acceptable practice.

DEFINITIONS OF MUCOSAL, SKIN, SOFT TISSUE, NERVE, AND BONE MARGINS

Another step toward improved communication of surgical margins lies in establishing working definitions. In mSCCa, definition of a 'positive' margin is variable and may include carcinoma at an inked margin,[2–4] tumor within 1 high-power field of an inked margin,[5] within 1 mm of an inked margin,[6] within 2 mm of an inked margin,[7] and inclusion of high-grade surface dysplasia and/or in situ carcinoma have also been described.[8] Failure to define the various 'types' of surgical margins that may undergo histologic evaluation and the manner in which they are sectioned/sampled[9,10] and examined may lead to interdisciplinary friction. The microscopic evaluation of the peripheral oral mucosal border around the resection specimen is often referred to as the 'mucosal' margin. A mucosal margin is not only composed of the surface epithelium, it invariably includes submucosal stroma, and very often superficial skeletal muscle

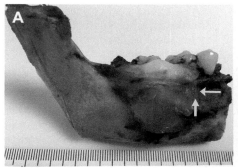
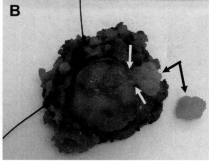

Fig. 2. Segmental mandibular resection performed for odontogenic myxoma exhibiting expansion through buccal cortical plate. Before inking, myxoid tissue grossly exposed at the lateral aspect of resection along the anterior border of the periosteal/bone interface (*white arrows*) and histologically confirmed as tumor. (*A*) Superficial parotidectomy specimen performed for management of pleomorphic adenoma. Two specimens noted in specimen cup (*black arrows*). Gross examination before inking reveals tumor extruded from defect area (between *white arrows*) in surgical specimen, and second small detached specimen also confirmed as tumor (*longer black arrow*) (*B*).

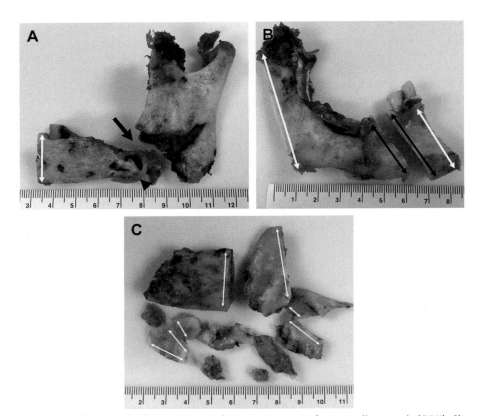

Fig. 3. Segmental mandibular resection performed for management of osteoradionecrosis (ORN). Site of pathologic fracture (*black arrow*) identified, inferior alveolar nerve (*arrowhead*), and area of planned bone margin evaluation spanned by *white line with arrows*. (*A*) Segmental mandibular resection performed for management of ORN. Two specimens included in same specimen cup, with larger portion representing initial resection and clinically suspicious nonviable anterior bone margin, resulting in same operation surgical revision. Surgeon confirms location of true bone margins (adjacent to *white line with arrows*) and opposing not-true surfaces (*black arrows*). (*B*) Multiple bone fragments in 1 specimen cup removed for management of ORN. Although multiple straight bone cuts present (*white line with arrows*), specimen fragmentation precludes confident identification of true bone margins (*C*).

bundles, nerve, or even salivary gland tissue, depending on the manner of specimen sampling, specimen size, and anatomic location. For resections involving skin, considerations for the 'skin' margins are similar to those of mucosal margins. The 'soft tissue' margins of a resection are composed of interstitial connective tissue, nerve, vascular channels, muscle, tendon and salivary tissue, essentially almost any tissue component with the exception of surface epithelial lining. A 'deep' margin indicates a specific orientation of a 'soft tissue' margin, although the term 'deep' margin is often used interchangeably with 'soft tissue' margin in a colloquial fashion (**Fig. 4**).

Transection of named nerves such as the lingual nerve may be tagged on the main specimen and evaluated specifically as '*named* nerve margin,' because this may represent a separate and unique path of possible tumor egress and margin

compromise. The surgeon may plan to revise a compromised named nerve and/or document areas of large nerve involvement for consideration of targeted adjuvant radiation therapy (**Fig. 5**). When a specimen margin (mucosal, soft tissue, nerve, bone or skin) is positive for neoplasm, it is important for the pathologist and surgeon to have clear communication regarding the anatomic location of the margin in relation to its harvested position from the specimen, and of equal importance is the *microscopic compartment* or level (surface epithelium, subepithelial lamina propria, muscle, etc) where the focus of carcinoma was detected for the surgeon to provide adequate size and volume of tissue, if revision of the compromised margin is under consideration (see **Fig. 1**D). Providing an intraoperative report of 'medial margin positive' is not sufficiently detailed for the surgeon to balance revision of a

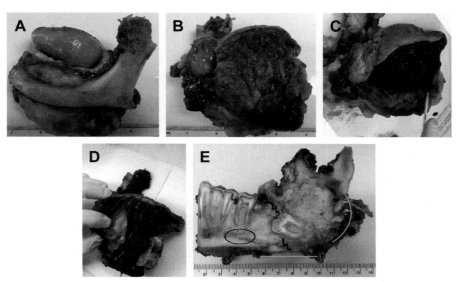

Fig. 4. Composite, segmental mandibular resection with hemiglossectomy and level I neck dissection performed for management of ventral tongue mucosal squamous cell carcinoma. Fresh resection specimen received at hand off (*A*), medial view (*B*), application of ink to mark medial/deep soft tissue margin. (*C*), perpendicular sections placed to evaluate tumor at closest approach to medial/deep soft tissue margin and (*D*) composite, segmental mandibular resection specimen (unrelated to case in *A–D*), sectioned in the sagittal plane after removal of mucosal margins, nerve margins, and formalin fixation. Neck contents removed and location inked (*blue line*) before sagittal sectioning. Closest soft tissue margin identified in this plane (*yellow*), region of anterior bone margin (*pink*), pathologic fracture (*black lightning bolts*), carcinoma extending anteriorly within mandibular canal (*black circle*) and gross invasion of masticator space musculature (*region of green semicircle*) supporting pathologic staging pT4b (*E*).

3-dimensional defect cavity with tissue conservation and function, unless the reported area coincides with a previously identified margin of concern by the surgeon.

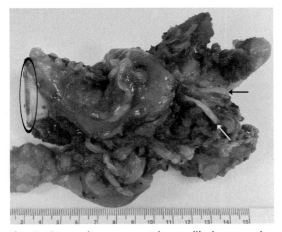

Fig. 5. Composite, segmental mandibular resection with in continuity neck contents performed in management of mucosal squamous cell carcinoma. V3 nerve stump before entering the mandibular canal (*black arrow*) and lingual nerve (*white arrow*) identified before nerve margin sampling. Anterior bone margin identified (*black circle*).

ARE ALL SURGICAL MARGINS EQUALLY IMPORTANT?

A resident trainee at recently queried whether mucosal margins were 'less important' than soft tissue, nerve, skin or bone margins. The perception of relative importance among margin tissue types (by surgeons or pathologists) might correlate with the areas most challenging to access intraoperatively, although institutional culture, inconsistent definitions, and/or underemphasis of specific margin reporting in the literature may also have a role.

Using oral mSCCa as a prototype disease, it has been suggested that surgeons are more likely to encounter difficulties in maintaining a safe barrier of uninvolved margin tissue in the deeper planes of the dissection when compared with the surgical placement of mucosal margins.[11] It follows then that the deeper soft tissue margins would be most frequently compromised when a positive margin is identified. One study of 301 patients with oral and oropharyngeal cancer noted that, in 70 patients with positive margins, the 'deep margin' was most commonly involved (87%; 61/70). Mucosal margins alone were uncommonly compromised (16%; 11/70) and 14% of cases (10/70) were identified as having a positive bone margin, although this was rarely in isolation.[12] Although this single study supports the notion that the deep margin is most *frequently* compromised when a positive margin is reported, no measure of importance can be assigned, and effects of other variables such as tumor size, location, previous treatment in the area, and variability in defining deep versus mucosal margins have not been adequately studied in the literature. Other investigators have suggested that smaller sized resections are more likely to have a compromised mucosal margin than a deep margin,[3] as the surgeon balances complete resection with tissue conservation, preservation of function, or approaches the limit of primary closure versus an expanding defect requiring free tissue reconstruction. Yuen and colleagues[13] identified submucosal microsatellite spread of oral tongue mSCCa (mucosal margin) almost as often as intramuscular (soft tissue margin) satellite spread of carcinoma (16% vs 22%, respectively), suggesting that, indeed, mucosal margins must be accurately sampled and evaluated.

A more systematic approach to the study of mSCCa surgical margins has been reported recently, with an emphasis on the source of margin tissue (resection specimen margins vs tumor bed margins) emerging as an important determinant of margin fidelity in the field of early stage oral mSCCa.[4,10,14,15] Margins sampled from the **tumor bed** are more likely to be mucosal margins, tend to be negative for neoplasm, show less correlation with final margin status of the final report, and with local recurrence.[4,14,15] Even on a molecular level, mucosal margins sampled from the tumor bed fail to correlate with local recurrence.[16] Similar to mucosal and soft tissue margins, Intra operative sampling of resection specimen-based bone margins more closely correlates with final bone margin status in contrast to tumor bed bone margin sampling.[17,18] Most studies of mSCCa do not specify whether the margins were sampled from the tumor bed, specimen resection, or both and few specify the margin type (mucosal, soft tissue, etc).[12,19–22] Increasing the level of detail reported for margin status may be more commonplace in future studies of mSCCa, as changes to the College of American Pathologists synoptic reporting guidelines to facilitate the reporting of margin status and source are now in place.[23,24]

In contrast to mucosal-based pathology, the margin evaluation of intraosseous gnathic tumors, such as ameloblastoma, tends to focus on the status of the bone margin(s).[25–27] Intact anatomic bone surfaces such as inferior border, medial, and lateral cortical bone are not subject to margin sampling. However when these bone surfaces are violated by tumor, the periosteal layer represents the next anatomic layer peripheral to the cortical bone, but can be attenuated or even breached by tumor. Although the literature emphasizes the status of the bone margins for intraosseous odontogenic neoplasms, the specimen mucosal, periosteal and/or soft tissue overlying bone defects, including initial biopsy site defects, requires the same attention to detail as given to bone margin analysis (**Fig. 6**). The dearth of studies on nonosseous resection margins for intraosseous neoplasms does not diminish the importance of this margin tissue type; ameloblastoma is known to recur in the bone or soft tissue.[28,29] In sum, because it remains challenging to correlate recurrent disease with a specific location or origin of a compromised margin, all surgical margins should be given equal consideration during the resection, and pathologic examination of margin tissue.

POSTREMOVAL SPECIMEN CHANGES

Similar to the query regarding relative margin importance, resident trainees have expressed uncertainty and/or concern that specimen shrinkage

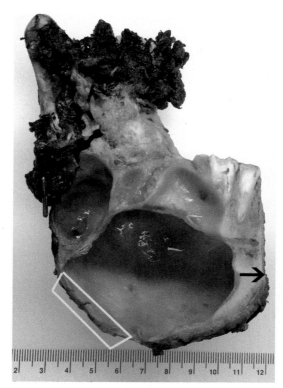

Fig. 6. Composite, segmental mandibular resection performed for the management of large ameloblastoma. Tumor invasion beyond cortical bone and overlying periosteum into adjacent soft tissue envelope represents closest soft tissue margin (*white box*). Arrow identifies closest bone margin.

encroaches on the safety margin excised surrounding mSCCa. This concept may in part be related to the manner in which measurements have been collected and compared. Studies evaluating postremoval changes have collected various measurements such as shrinkage of the tumor, shrinkage of the overall specimen size, or shrinkage of the linear dimension between the clinically visible tumor and the cut margin.[30] Tumor shrinkage is known to occur and alterations in tumor size can impact accurate staging of any tumor staged by size; therefore, the surgeon and the pathology team should carefully document the borders, dimensions, and measurement of the tumor, particularly at the cutoff points of 2 and 4 cm in the fresh resection specimen.[21,31] Shrinkage of the overall specimen size may become problematic in certain excisions requiring the billing of surgical procedures by size, most often in cutaneous surgery, given the appearance of discordant measurements.[32]

Data collection of mSCCa margin shrinkage has variably included measurements of the **in vivo** margin measurement (the linear distance between the border of clinically evident mucosal lesion to the planned site of the peripheral 'mucosal' margin as marked with a tissue marking pen before resection), the fresh, **unfixed ex vivo** margin measurement (the linear distance between the border of clinically evident mucosal lesion to the now-cut peripheral 'mucosal' margin of the specimen), and the postfixation, or **in vitro** margin measurement (the linear distance between the border of clinically evident mucosal lesion to the peripheral 'mucosal' margin of the specimen after variable time spent in formalin fixation).[33–36] These **clinically** based tumor-to-margin measurements obtained with rulers or calipers are then compared with *histologic* measurements of tumor islands to the closest inked margin, as measured with a microscope. There has been little control of confounding elements, such pattern of tumor invasion, location of the histologic measurement(s) relative to the initial clinical measurement, and variability in personnel obtaining measurements in the clinical versus laboratory conditions. An attempt to calculate the difference between clinical measurements of surface findings and the histologic measurements of submucosal measurements as percent margin shrinkage in mSCCa seems discordant and more rigorous study in this field, in addition to the study of other neoplastic processes, is required.

INDETERMINATE RESECTION MARGIN STATUS

The rate of indeterminate margin status is reported to range between 4% to 20% in mSCCa.[37,38] Few papers report their experience or rate of indeterminate margin status, which limits understanding of the factors or circumstances that undermine confident margin assessment. Anecdotal scenarios are available related to surgical variables (intraoperative gross tumor fragmentation, marked procedural artifacts including cautery), pathology-related variables (dissection/sectioning of inadvertently uninked specimen, physical dislodgement, and loss of margin tissue during frozen section analysis or from a formalin-fixed paraffin block),[39] and/or related to communication, such as receipt of unoriented, multipart resection specimens received in formalin, all containing tumor that cannot be related grossly or microscopically, to one another (**Fig. 7**). In rare instances, unusual

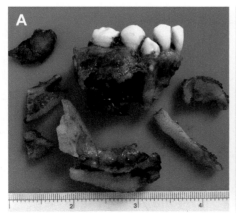
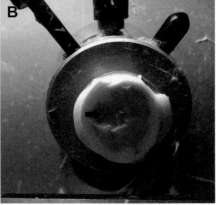

Fig. 7. Segmental mandibular resection performed for the management of mandibular ameloblastoma. Multiple specimen fragments received in 1 formalin-filled specimen cup precludes accurate margin status reporting (*A*). Portion of margin tissue being evaluated at frozen section displaced (*black arrow*) by microtome cutting blade, precluding margin reporting. Surgeon notified intraoperatively and revised margin submitted for examination (*B*).

tumor related variables, such as finding lympho-vascular invasion crossing an inked margin, or abundant free mucin at an inked margin in resection of mucoepidermoid carcinoma, or bland appearing 'adipose' tissue extending to an inked margin in well-differentiated liposarcoma, may present as problematic for margin reporting.

Aside from surgical resection specimens that preclude margin reporting, such as surgical gross total resection or resection specimen fragmentation, the pathologist and surgeon should maintain open communication to attempt to accurately resolve a possible indeterminate margin scenario. Review of the handoff notes and gross examination, any photographs, and correlation with the residual specimen may be helpful in some cases, depending on circumstances. In cases where margin tissue is submitted in multiple separate specimen cups, which increases complexity in margin reconciliation, the most recent College of American Pathologists guidelines may be helpful.[22] External pathology review/second opinion consultation is limited almost exclusively to diagnostic classification, not adjudication of margin status, and therefore unlikely to be a fruitful resource, particularly when the gross examination descriptions are inadequate, the method of sampling (shave vs radial), or the intent of the sampling mechanism (incisional biopsy vs excision) is unclear.[40,41] There is very little literature to guide pathologists, surgeons, or subsequent treating physicians in the head and neck multidisciplinary team regarding this difficult and poorly described challenge in patient care, and therefore where possible, prevention of indeterminate margin status is critical.

SUMMARY

The ability to correlate study results and surgical margins within a disease type is impeded by variability in operational definitions, and the inclusion of patients with a spectrum of disease sites, stages, and putative histopathologic prognostic variables, among others. Margin tissue may be composed of multiple different tissue types, and the microscopic tissue location, in addition to the gross anatomic location of a compromised margin, is important information to enable successful revision where revision is desirable. Reporting of surgical margin conditions in the literature, although recently improved, is still lacking in overall detail. The number of positive margins, tissue type, number of attempts at intraoperative revision versus revision by second procedure, and resolving difficult-to-define concepts ('focal' positive margin) await future study.

ACKNOWLEDGMENTS

The author wishes to acknowledge and thank Simon I. Chiosea, MD for his expertise, suggestions and thoughtful review of this manuscript.

REFERENCES

1. Black C, Marotti J, Zarovnaya E, et al. Critical evaluation of frozen section margins in head and neck cancer resections. Cancer 2006;107(12):2792–800.
2. Patel RS, Goldstein DP, Guillemaud J, et al. Impact of positive frozen section microscopic tumor cut-through revised to negative on oral carcinoma control and survival rates. Head Neck 2010;32(11):1444–51.
3. Scholl P, Byers RM, Batsakis JG, et al. Microscopic cut-through of cancer in the surgical treatment of squamous carcinoma of the tongue. Prognostic and therapeutic implications. Am J Surg 1986; 152(4):354–60.
4. Maxwell JH, Thompson LD, Brandwein-Gensler MS, et al. Early oral tongue squamous cell carcinoma: sampling of margins from tumor bed and worse local control. JAMA Otolaryngol Head Neck Surg 2015;141:1–8.
5. Spiro RH, Guillamondegui O Jr, Paulino AF, et al. Pattern of invasion and margin assessment in patients with oral tongue cancer. Head Neck 1999; 21(5):408–13.
6. Woolgar JA. Histopathological prognosticators in oral and oropharyngeal squamous cell carcinoma. Oral Oncol 2006;42(3):229–39.
7. Pathak KA, Nason RW, Penner C, et al. Impact of use of frozen section assessment of operative margins on survival in oral cancer. Oral Surg Oral Med Oral Pathol Oral Radiol Endod 2009; 107(2):235–9.
8. Batsakis JG. Surgical excision margins: a pathologist's perspective. Adv Anat Pathol 1999;6(3):140–8.
9. Williams MD. Determining adequate margins in head and neck cancers: practice and continued challenges. Curr Oncol Rep 2016;18(9):54.
10. Chiosea SI. Intraoperative margin assessment in early oral squamous cell carcinoma. Surg Pathol Clin 2017;10(1):1–14.
11. Hinni ML, Ferlito A, Brandwein-Gensler MS, et al. Surgical margins in head and neck cancer: a contemporary review. Head Neck 2013;35(9):1362–70.
12. Woolgar JA, Triantafyllou A. A histopathological appraisal of surgical margins in oral and oropharyngeal cancer resection specimens. Oral Oncol 2005; 41(10):1034–43.
13. Yuen PW, Lam KY, Chan AC, et al. Clinicopathological analysis of local spread of carcinoma of the tongue. Am J Surg 1998;175(3):242–4.
14. Chang AM, Kim SW, Duvvuri U, et al. Early squamous cell carcinoma of the oral tongue: comparing

margins obtained from the glossectomy specimen to margins from the tumor bed. Oral Oncol 2013; 49(11):1077–82.

15. Yahalom R, Dobriyan A, Vered M, et al. A prospective study of surgical margin status in oral squamous cell carcinoma: a preliminary report. J Surg Oncol 2008;98(8):572–8.

16. Huang X, Pateromichelakis S, Hills A, et al. p53 mutations in deep tissues are more strongly associated with recurrence than mutation-positive mucosal margins. Clin Cancer Res 2007;13(20):6099–106.

17. Mahmood S, Conway D, Ramesar KC. Use of intra-operative cytologic assessment of mandibular marrow scrapings to predict resection margin status in patients with squamous cell carcinoma. J Oral Maxillofac Surg 2001;59(10):1138–41.

18. Bilodeau EA, Chiosea S. Oral squamous cell carcinoma with mandibular bone invasion: intraoperative evaluation of bone margins by routine frozen section. Head Neck Pathol 2011;5(3):216–20.

19. Sutton DN, Brown JS, Rogers SN, et al. The prognostic implications of the surgical margin in oral squamous cell carcinoma. Int J Oral Maxillofac Surg 2003;32(1):30–4.

20. Loree TR, Strong EW. Significance of positive margins in oral cavity squamous carcinoma. Am J Surg 1990; 160(4):410–4.

21. Hicks WL Jr, North JH Jr, Loree TR, et al. Surgery as a single modality therapy for squamous cell carcinoma of the oral tongue. Am J Otolaryngol 1998; 19(1):24–8.

22. Sieczka E, Datta R, Singh A, et al. Cancer of the buccal mucosa: are margins and T-stage accurate predictors of local control? Am J Otolaryngol 2001; 22(6):395–9.

23. Amin MB, Edge SB, Greene FL, et al. AJCC cancer staging manual. 8th edition. Chicago: Springer; 2017.

24. College of American Pathologists. Protocol for the examination of specimens from patients with carcinomas of the lip and oral cavity. 2016. Available at: http://www.cap.org/ShowProperty?nodePath=/UCMCon/Contribution%20Folders/WebContent/pdf/liporalcaversion-16protocol.pdf. Accessed May 16, 2017.

25. De Silva I, Rozen WM, Ramakrishnan A, et al. Achieving adequate margins in ameloblastoma resection: the role for intra-operative specimen imaging. Clinical report and systematic review. PLoS One 2012;7(10):e47897.

26. Kalaiselvan S, Dharmesh Kumar Raja AV, Saravanan B, et al. "Evaluation of safety margin" in ameloblastoma of the mandible by surgical, radiological, and histopathological methods: an evidence-based study. J Pharm Bioallied Sci 2016;8(Suppl 1): S122–5.

27. Peacock ZS, Ji YD, Faquin WC. What is important for confirming negative margins when resecting mandibular ameloblastomas? J Oral Maxillofac Surg 2017;75(6):1185–90.

28. Yang R, Liu Z, Peng C, et al. Maxillary ameloblastoma: factors associated with risk of recurrence. Head Neck 2017;39(5):996–1000.

29. Daramola JO, Ajagbe HA, Oluwasanmi JO. Recurrent ameloblastoma of the jaws–a review of 22 cases. Plast Reconstr Surg 1980;65(5):577–9.

30. Chen CH, Hsu MY, Jiang RS, et al. Shrinkage of head and neck cancer specimens after formalin fixation. J Chin Med Assoc 2012;75(3):109–13.

31. Brotherston D, Poon I, Peerani R, et al. Tumor shrinkage associated with whole-mount histopathologic techniques in oral tongue carcinoma. Pathol Res Pract 2015;211(5):398–403.

32. Dauendorffer JN, Bastuji-Garin S, Guero S, et al. Shrinkage of skin excision specimens: formalin fixation is not the culprit. Br J Dermatol 2009;160(4): 810–4.

33. Pangare TB, Waknis PP, Bawane SS, et al. Effect of formalin fixation on surgical margins in patients with oral squamous cell carcinoma. J Oral Maxillofac Surg 2017;75(6):1293–8.

34. Mistry RC, Qureshi SS, Kumaran C. Post-resection mucosal margin shrinkage in oral cancer: quantification and significance. J Surg Oncol 2005;91(2):131–3.

35. Johnson RE, Sigman JD, Funk GF, et al. Quantification of surgical margin shrinkage in the oral cavity. Head Neck 1997;19(4):281–6.

36. Cheng A, Cox D, Schmidt BL. Oral squamous cell carcinoma margin discrepancy after resection and pathologic processing. J Oral Maxillofac Surg 2008;66(3):523–9.

37. Ransohoff A, Wood D, Solomon Henry A, et al. Third party assessment of resection margin status in head and neck cancer. Oral Oncol 2016;57:27–31.

38. de Almeida JR, Li R, Magnuson JS, et al. Oncologic outcomes after transoral robotic surgery: a multi-institutional study. JAMA Otolaryngol Head Neck Surg 2015;141(12):1043–51.

39. Blasdale C, Charlton FG, Weatherhead SC, et al. Effect of tissue shrinkage on histological tumour-free margin after excision of basal cell carcinoma. Br J Dermatol 2010;162(3):607–10.

40. Westra WH, Kronz JD, Eisele DW. The impact of second opinion surgical pathology on the practice of head and neck surgery: a decade experience at a large referral hospital. Head Neck 2002;24(7):684–93.

41. Zhu GA, Lira R, Colevas AD. Discordance in routine second opinion pathology review of head and neck oncology specimens: a single-center five year retrospective review. Oral Oncol 2016;53:36–41.

Margin Analysis—Has Free Tissue Transfer Improved Oncologic Outcomes for Oral Squamous Cell Carcinoma?

Sean P. Edwards, MD, DDS, FRCD(C)[a,b,*]

KEYWORDS

- Microvascular tissue transfer • Free flaps • Surgical margins • Oncologic outcomes
- Oral squamous cell carcinoma

KEY POINTS

- Free tissue transfer is a reliable, safe method of reconstruction of defects of the head and neck.
- Negative surgical margins improve locoregional tumor control.
- Despite trends for improved oncologic outcomes with free tissue transfer, there are no conclusive data within the published literature to validate this statement.

A former tenet of head and neck surgery was that the ablative procedure should never be dictated by a surgeon's reconstructive skills. Taken a step further, some units divided the ablative and reconstructive teams to avoid compromising a resection in an effort to match a given reconstructive plan. When a reconstructive armamentarium is limited to local and regional flaps, tissue volume and component options are limited. Simple human nature dictates being more conservative with the margins that are sought to be achieved. Free tissue transfer offers myriad options in terms of volume and character of tissue that may be used to reconstruct virtually any head and neck defect. Without a doubt, most surgeons admit taking wider margins when a decision has been made to proceed with a free tissue reconstruction.

Surgical margin status is frequently reported to be a strong predictor of outcome and this remains, at least to some degree, partly under the control of the surgeon as a technical exercise.[1,2] When attempting to examine whether the use of free tissue transfer has a relationship with oncologic outcome investigators have approached this question from this angle: Freed from reconstructive constraints to take any surgical margin desired, will oncologic outcomes improve? That said, when reviewing the potential impact of free tissue transfer on oncologic outcomes, the following elements should be considered.

First, regarding margins, does free tissue transfer result in wider margins? This seems not always to be the case. Ellis and colleagues[3] examined the records of 250 patients treated for oral cavity cancer that were not able to show that surgeons achieved wider margins when free flaps were used. By contrast, Hanosono and colleagues[4] found their rate of positive margins dropped from

No relevant financial disclosures.

[a] Oral and Maxillofacial Surgery Residency Program, University of Michigan, 1500 E Medical Center Drive RM C213, Ann Arbor, MI 48109, USA; [b] Pediatric Maxillofacial Surgery, C.S. Mott Children's Hospital, Michigan Medicine, 1540 E Hospital Drive SPC 4219, Ann Arbor, MI 48109-4219, USA

* Corresponding author. Oral and Maxillofacial Surgery Residency Program, University of Michigan, 1500 E Medical Center Drive RM C213, Ann Arbor, MI.

E-mail address: seanedwa@med.umich.edu

Oral Maxillofacial Surg Clin N Am 29 (2017) 377–381
http://dx.doi.org/10.1016/j.coms.2017.05.001

18% to 7% with the introduction of free tissue transfer to their unit. It is hard to imagine that surgeons are not more liberal with margins when reliable free tissue transfer options are at their disposal but it is also likely true that margin status is a reflection of tumor biology and, in this regard, something beyond the control of the surgeon.

Second, it should be considered that given the overall reliability of free tissue transfer, with success rates routinely in excess of 90%, it is possible that these patients will more reliably receive on-time adjuvant therapy and thereby enjoy a survival benefit. It is also possible that the functional gains achieved with free tissue transfer lead to better health and nutrition of patients that may also have an impact on survival. This is a complex issue.

How then would this question ideally be studied? Because of the indisputable benefits of free tissue transfer on reconstructive grounds, it is unethical to design a study where patients are randomized to an inferior reconstructive option. As such, most efforts in this regard rely on historical data, making robust comparisons challenging. This introduces significant potential for bias. If modern era outcomes were compared with those of the past, any changes seen would be the aggregate of improved patient selection, medical care, and adjuvant care in addition to frank changes in disease patterns, such as the rise in prevalence of human papillomavirus–related disease. Surrogate lines of inquiry could instead focus on factors believed associated with better oncologic outcomes, such as the frequency of on-time delivery of adjuvant chemoradiotherapy.

Consider an indirect comparison. Marchetti and colleagues[5] compared a retrospective series of 42 consecutively treated oral cavity cancers to 3 historical series from the pre–free flap era spanning the late 1950s to the early 1980s. The investigators' series include T2 through T4 tumors all treated with resection and microvascular reconstruction. They offer few operative data from this patient population other than oral cavity subsite and TNM staging. Unfortunately, the investigators did not include margin status from their resections. As discussed previously, such a comparison is weak at best with significant potential for bias and errors in the comparison. With that in mind, the investigators were not able to demonstrate a difference in survival for patients in their study compared with the historical samples.

Direct comparisons reduce some of the potential for bias because the patient populations are potentially more similar. The investigators (discussed later) conducted single-institution reviews of their patient populations and used a variety of methods to attempt to glean useful information from the differences in treatment therein.

Rogers and colleagues[6] conducted a retrospective review of a consecutive series of 489 oral cavity cancer patients treated over a 10-year period; 65% of their patients received a free flap as part of their treatment. On a univariate analysis, free flap surgery was associated with a worse overall (72% vs 51%) and disease-specific (88% vs 70%) 5-year survival. Importantly there was no effort to match patients by factors known to affect outcome, so it is likely this is a reflection of higher-stage disease. In support of this, free flap surgery was not found an independent predictor of disease-specific survival when analyzed as part of a multivariable Cox regression analysis (hazard ratio 0.9). In further support of this assertion, the same pattern was seen for radiotherapy in this study in that it was associated with worse survival on univariate analysis but not when analyzed as part of a multivariable Cox regression analysis (hazard ratio 0.8).

Hsieh and colleagues[7] sought to be more selective when studying this question and focused on patients with late-stage disease. Specifically, this group analyzed the impact of free tissue transfer in a cohort of patients from a single Taiwanese institution treated between 2002 and 2008 with stage IV oral squamous cell carcinoma. No patient had evidence of distant disease. In their sample, 93 patients underwent free flap reconstruction and 149 patients did not due to limited defects, poor-quality recipient vessels, and/or significant medical comorbidities. The medical exclusions in the non–free flap group accounted for only 3% of the patients (n = 4/149). All patients were followed for at least 18 months or until death. When comparing the 2 groups, they were similar in most features except that the free flap group presented with larger tumors, more buccal lesions, fewer tongue cancers, and more T4 tumors (66% vs 50%) than the non–free flap group. When analyzing outcomes between the 2 groups, the investigators found a nonsignificant trend to a lower incidence of positive margins of 17.2% versus 12.1% (P = .213). Further comparisons did not find any significant differences in recurrence rates, local recurrence rates, 5-year overall survival, and 5 year disease-specific survival. Although the investigators highlight that the free flap group had similar survival despite more advanced T stage, it is hard to draw a definitive conclusion about oncologically superior outcomes with free flaps in this study.

Hanasono and colleagues[4] completed a 25-year retrospective review of all patients with T3 and T4 disease surgically resected at the MD Anderson Cancer Center. At this center, microsurgical techniques were incorporated after 1989. This allowed the investigators to develop 2 cohorts. The non-microsurgical cohort comprised 135 patients treated between 1980 and 1989 and, of those, 63 patients in this group underwent some form of non-microsurgical reconstruction. The microsurgical free flap group included 231 patients treated after the year 1989. Demographically the 2 groups were similar except for an increased incidence of hypertension and diabetes in the post-1989 cohort as well as an increase in the T and N stages. Therapeutically, the latter group has a higher rate of adjuvant therapy, 52% versus 69% for radiation therapy and 2% versus 18% for chemotherapy. The latter group was also more likely to have a received a selective neck dissection instead of a modified radical neck dissection. The investigators then compared the 2 groups in reference to the incidence of positive margins, recurrence, and survival at 3 years and 5 years. The investigators found no difference in overall survival, disease-specific survival, disease-free interval, and locoregional recurrence rates despite more advanced T and N stages in the 1989 to 2004 group. The only significant difference between the 2 groups was the incidence of positive margins, which decreased in the post-1989 sample from 18% to 7% (**Fig. 1**).

De Vicente and colleagues[8] undertook a retrospective review of a cohort of 98 patients treated in a single unit over a 20-year period. All patients had a primary oral squamous cell carcinoma, staged as T2 or greater, resected with frozen section control and neck dissection. Half of the patients had a formal free flap reconstruction with the remainder receiving local and/or regional flaps. The latter (no free flap) group was randomly selected and stage-matched from the time period prior to the introduction of free tissue transfer in this unit. Radiotherapy was delivered to those who were pT4 and had regional nodal disease or a positive margin. The investigators defined 2 clinical endpoints, death from disease recurrence or nontreatable disease at the end of the follow-up period. The investigators make no mention of using these for a sample size calculation. The groups were well matched in terms of demographics, tumor features, and adjuvant treatment rates, with a significant difference noted only in that the free flap group had a greater number of patients under the age of 60 years. At the end of the follow-up period, a statistically significant difference in survival was noted between the 2 groups using the Fisher exact test but not using univariate Kaplan-Meier analysis. The microvascular group had a 53% disease-specific survival rate whereas the locoregional flap control group suffered a 33% survival rate. The free flap group had mean and median survival times of 65 months and 60 months, respectively, whereas the corresponding times in the control sample were 54 months and 24 months, respectively. There was no difference in the incidence of positive margins between the 2 groups. Margin status was significantly associated with survival in the group as a whole and in the free flap group (**Fig. 2**).

In these studies, there seems to be a trend to better survival with either longer periods of time to recurrence or equivalent survival rates despite more advanced disease. The samples sizes in these reviews are small and are likely too small to detect a difference at a statistically significant level.

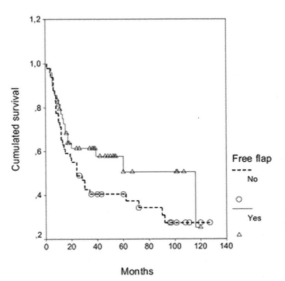

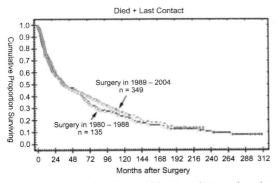

Fig. 1. Survival of patients with T3 and T4 oral cavity cancers after surgical treatment. The 1980 to 1988 line represents the pre–free flap cohort and the 1989 to 2004 line is the cohort where free flaps were used.

Fig. 2. Kaplan-Meier survival analysis shows nonsignificant trend to better survival and longer survival time despite no difference in margin status, staging, and therapy.

The best evidence in support of the oncologic benefits of free tissue transfer comes from Mucke and colleagues.[9] These investigators undertook a single-institution, retrospective chart review of 773 patient with oral squamous cell carcinoma treated over a 14-year period. The initial chart review included 1237 patients. Excluded from this number were those with nonoral squamous cell carcinoma, synchronous tumors, close or positive margins, and persistent disease defined as recurrence within 6 months. It is unfortunate the investigators chose to exclude those with close or positive because differences here may reflect a behavioral change on the part of ablative surgeons when microsurgical reconstructive techniques are available. Dependent variables for analysis were overall survival at 5 years and survival in months.

Demographic and disease characteristics were similar between the 2 groups except for a trend to higher T stage and N stage and tumor grade in the free flap group. The 5-year survival for their entire cohort was 61.4% with a mean survival time of 67.6 months. For those not receiving a free flap, 5-year survival and mean survival time was measured as 58.8% and 66.8 months, respectively. This was poorer than the cohort of 274 patients who received a free flap where 5-year survival was 66.2% and mean survival time was 69.0 months. Under both univariate and multivariate analysis, microsurgical reconstruction was strongly associated with increased survival (**Fig. 3**). A further analysis of this cohort consisted of a matched pair analysis wherein a random matching of patients was accomplished based on T stage, N stage, histologic grade, and patient age. This was then subjected to Cox proportional hazard regression model analysis. A total of 256 patients in the free flap group was matched. Again,

immediate free flap reconstruction was significantly associated with survival, with a hazard ratio of 0.58 ($P<.001$). As expected, patient age, T stage, and N stage were also associated with survival whereas histologic grade was not.

As discussed previously, a significant flaw in the study by Mucke and colleagues[9] involves the failure to analyze those patients with positive and close margins, because it is widely believed that margin status is not only indicative of the quality of the resection but also the biology of the disease. By censuring the cohort to those with clear surgical margins, the study results cannot exclude biologically less aggressive disease as a confounding variable, resulting in sample bias. That said, the investigators demonstrated a clear trend to better survival that was seen on univariate and multivariate analysis of the whole sample and again in matched pair analysis.

Free tissue transfer has been widely adopted in most head and neck units for primary reconstruction of ablative defects of the head and neck because of its excellent reliability and the improvements it offers in terms of esthetics, function, and quality of life. Several investigators have attempted to answer the question of whether or not free tissue transfer has contributed to improved oncologic outcomes in head and neck cancer. As discussed previously, this is a difficult question to study but it is safe to conclude that outcomes have not suffered with its routine application and there may be a trend to improved survival with such contemporary reconstructive techniques. Survival in head and neck cancer is and will always be a composite outcome informed by disease biology, quality of surgery and adjuvant therapy, and potentially the quality of the reconstruction. The benefits of free tissue transfer in this patient population are indisputable even if it cannot be said with certainty that they have improved oncologic outcomes.

REFERENCES

1. Luryi AL, Chen MM, Mehra S, et al. Positive surgical margins in early stage oral cavity cancer: an analysis of 20,602 cases. Otolaryngol Head Neck Surg 2014; 151:984–90.
2. Sutton DN, Brown JS, Rogers SN, et al. The prognostic implications of the surgical margin in oral squamous cell carcinoma. Int J Oral Maxillofac Surg 2003; 32:30–4.
3. Ellis OG, David MC, Park DJ, et al. High volume surgeons deliver larger surgical margins in oral cavity cancer. J Oral Maxillofac Surg 2016;74:1466–72.
4. Hanasono MM, Friel MT, Klem C, et al. Impact of reconstructive microsurgery in patients with

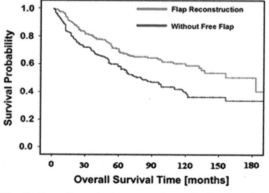

Fig. 3. Overall survival curves of matched pairs. Flap reconstruction was associated with statistically significant improvement in survival.